G000043706

Fats Nutrition and Health

Fats Nutrition and Health

The complete guide to what fats are, what they do, and what makes them healthy or harmful

ROBERT ERDMANN Ph.D.
and MEIRION JONES

THORSONS PUBLISHING GROUP

First published in 1990

© Robert Erdmann and Meirion Jones 1990

*All rights reserved. No part of this book may be reproduced or utilized in any form or by
any means, electronic or mechanical, including photocopying, recording or by any
information storage and retrieval system, without permission in writing from the Publisher.*

British Library Cataloguing in Publication Data

Erdmann, Robert
Fats, Nutrition and health.
1. Man. Nutrition. Role of fats
I. Title   II. Jones, Meirion
613.2'8

ISBN 0 7225 1962 1

Published by Thorsons Publishers Limited,
Wellingborough, Northamptonshire, NN8 2RQ, England

Typeset by Harper Phototypesetters Limited, Northampton, England
Printed in Great Britain by Mackays of Chatham, Kent

1 3 5 7 9 10 8 6 4 2

Contents

Introduction

A short walk from my practice in Tunbridge Wells stands one of the new breed of superstore, an enormous red-brick structure capped by four floors of car park. In the summer of 1988, my wife and I were shopping there when we noticed a woman dressed in a spotless imitation of a milkmaid's outfit, distributing samples of a new 'low-fat spread' to passing shoppers. As we approached, I heard her describing the merits of the spread to a couple of attentive consumers. Spreading a little of the product onto some meagre quarters of cracker, she emphasized repeatedly that it was better for their health than butter since it was 'high in polyunsaturates and low in saturates and fat'. She pronounced these words mechanically as if she wasn't absolutely sure what they meant.

Intrigued, I asked her what a polyunsaturate was, and why it made the product worth buying. She shrugged and produced a sheaf of briefing notes from behind her counter. 'Perhaps it means it spreads more easily,' she suggested. I asked her why an easier spread was better for my health. 'I know I can't explain very clearly but I expect most people know what a polyunsaturate is,' she replied, her tone suggesting that I was being troublesome.

I turned to the two shoppers and asked each in turn if they knew. Neither did. 'You know something about it, don't you?' said one of them to me. 'Tell us what it is.' So I did, explaining about the carbon chains of fatty acids and how they are either occupied fully with hydrogen atoms – making them saturated – or lacking a certain number of hydrogen atoms – making them unsaturated. Not surprisingly, their faces glazed over. When I finished, I asked if the fact that the spread was high in polyunsaturates would make them buy it. One said yes: 'the important thing is that it's low in fat,' she said. 'Am I right?'

By now the curiosity bug had bitten me. Intrigued at what people know, and think they know, about fat, I stood at the exit of the shop for an hour the following afternoon conducting a fat *vox pop*. 'Butter makes you fat; margarine is good for you.' 'Fat builds up in your heart.' 'Fat is turned into starch.' 'No, I don't know what a polyunsaturate is . . . I buy X . . . why? . . . because its got polyunsaturates in it.' 'Fat is a poison.' These responses were both illuminating and disturbing.

Fat is food

My work with nutritional supplementation involves helping people to realize and exploit the enormous health-enhancing potential of good nutrition. I try to make people conscious of the fact that whatever they eat profoundly affects everything they are and do. Here, though, outside a food market in a country that claims to have some of the highest food quality standards in the world, people were revealing how little they associate their food with their well-being. Almost righteously they were buying food – such as these high-in-polyunsaturate margarines – on the strength of brazenly misapplied scientific terms with no clear idea of their meaning.

There was one thing they were clear about, though, and that was the idea that fat is a substance to be feared. It is associated in people's minds with cardio-vascular disease, cancer and impotence, not to mention its unpleasant physical appearance. The scientific terms, it seems, are merely a clever marketing gimmick to exploit the fear.

So how well-founded is this fear of fat? Is fat of any practical use to the body? When working with patients, my efforts are centred on helping them to overcome illness and debility by supplying in optimum amounts all the nutrients that are essential to the body and which, judging by the illness, may be lacking. These include vitamins (vitamin C, B complex and so on), minerals (zinc, magnesium and selenium plus others), and essential amino acids (the unadulterated building blocks of protein). I also use fats. Some shoppers might blanch but not only do I use them, I sometimes administer them in very high quantities. I do this because they are every bit as important to the body as any other food you can name.

I know fats as something other than the commonly advanced view of them as dietary demons. I know certain fats as essential components of cell structure and metabolism – transmitting nerve messages, dictating behaviour and

8

participating in millions of reactions that are essential for health and vitality. There are many varieties of fat and each perform different functions. Some are inert, sitting in the body like unwanted baggage. Others are among the most biochemically active substances on earth. Fats cause the trouble they do because, thanks to food processing, refining, unbalanced diets and sedentary lifestyles, the inert fats have come to predominate over the active varieties. Man has made of fat an enemy instead of a valued friend. Therefore, to live at maximum potential and vitality that friendship should be reforged. That is where this book comes in.

In *Fats, Nutrition and Health*, our aim is to explain clearly what fat is and how it works in the body. We examine the different factors that have turned fat against us – why it is associated with so many illnesses and diseases – and how things can be set right. This book looks at the different sorts of fat to be found in the ordinary diet and which foods to eat to increase your intake of the good varieties. Once and for all the meaning of the terms saturate and unsaturate will be explained, together with other terms often heard but rarely understood. We will see how food processing ravages dietary essential fat, what fats are the best ones to cook with and how to tell the difference between butter and margarine. More than anything else, this book will serve as a foundation to show you how to use certain fats actively and confidently to improve your health and actually to help reduce weight.

If you think that is a paradox, then read on.

Bob Erdmann

Part One

Elementary Fats

Chapter 1

Face the Fats

Imagine a book on the technique of a great master painter, so narrow in scope that it is concerned solely with the use of one colour from the many he applies to his canvases. Very quickly, the art historian reading the book realizes that no matter how well the artist's subtle application of that colour is conjured to life, no matter how evocative the description of the delicate brushwork, neither the painting nor the book makes sense. This is hardly surprising, since it is impossible to visualize the colour without thinking in terms of the painting as a whole. To make sense of its subject, the book will need to drop such extreme specialization and pull back to look at the broader canvas. Only by seeing how this colour complements the others in the paintings, how it adds dramatic highlight, perhaps, how it is blended on the palette to suggest space and depth, will the subject be understood.

Of course books with titles like *Rubens and Yellow Ochre* or *Van Gogh: The Red Connection* suggest such an impossibly narrow genre that they will never be published. Yet, time and again, books appear on health and nutrition which make a similar mistake, focusing so intently on one preferred substance or another, one illness, or on one supposed miracle therapy, that the positions of these factors in the overall functions of the body seem to be forgotten.

Despite apparent evidence to the contrary – in women's magazines and diet books, advertising campaigns for low-fat dairy produce and substitutes and so-called calorie-controlled diets – fat isn't a subject that can be conveniently isolated. It doesn't sit in the body like an aloof train passenger ignoring his fellow travellers. On the contrary, it is an integral part of the body's dynamic, constantly evolving organic mechanism and for fat to be understood this point has to be appreciated.

Therefore, if we want to improve our health by altering our fat intake –

changing the sort of fat we eat or cutting down overall – it's vital to grasp the role that fat plays in the body. This book will be looking at fat in depth, examining its constituents, what use the body makes of it, and how good fats and bad will affect health. It will detail the way that fat is changed, often detrimentally, by processing, how certain fat-based nutritional supplements can help improve overall health, and the best ways of cooking with fat. But it will do this by constantly relating back to fat's role in the bodily functions. Under the circumstances, a good place for us to start is to see just what that role is.

Fat and the metabolic treadmill

In common with all foods, fats are used in what are called metabolic pathways.[1] These are cyclic chemical reactions that custom-build for the body every single substance – enzymes, hormones, hair, teeth, muscles, eyes, organs, blood and bones – that it needs in order to live. Metabolic pathways also help to break down and dispose of dead and exhausted tissue. Some of this will then be used in other reactions to create different structures and chemicals; the rest will be excreted. Since there is a limit to the variety of food substances available to us to eat and drink, the first action of the metabolic pathways is to dismantle the food, tearing it apart in the gut into its constituent molecules, distributing these throughout the body via the liver and circulatory system, and then refashioning them to exactly the form needed. Since metabolic pathways are an incredibly complicated, self-sustaining continuum, the molecules may well be reconstructed as enzymes which will in turn be used to break down other food molecules.

The need for metabolic pathways becomes clear just by looking at what we eat. Although a substance such as protein is used widely in our bodies, this is not to say that, for example, the flesh from the chicken leg I had for lunch – itself a good protein source – could be used to make a section of my eyes or hair, fitting it in as easily as a window frame can be lifted from a demolished house and fitted into another. Rather, the flesh must be digested and broken down into its constituents – amino acids, vitamins, minerals, carbohydrates and fats. Certain of these constituents will then be circulated to the eye cells and reassembled in a different form together with necessary substances obtained from other foods. This process requires hormones to control the process and enzymes to tear apart and rebuild and, of course, these chemicals are made by metabolic pathways, too.[2]

Metabolic pathways are, in effect, biochemical production lines whose seemingly endless chemical interactions and products provide us with the vital substances of life. Since everything we eat, and every chemical in our bodies, is related to every other like the members of an extended family tree, it is impossible to write about fats without including the actions of other nutrients. Here are some examples. They will be dealt with in more depth later but they give a good feel as to how closely interrelated fat is.

1. Inside every cell, tiny biochemical factories are generating thousands of new protein molecules every minute. To ensure that this production is executed smoothly, that only those molecules the body needs are produced, and that it doesn't create too many, the body produces hormones. These are biochemical 'supervisors' which oversee the process. Hormones include substances such as thyroxin and certain steroids to control growth; prostaglandins which, amongst other things, regulate our immune response to viral infection; and oestrogen, which determines the body's fertility in women. Each of these, and many more, are made mainly from fat.[3]

2. The way that messages are passed from nerve cell to nerve cell makes another good example. These messages are responsible for all the body's mechanical activity, such as ordering the heart to beat, muscles to contract or mouth to salivate. The electrical impulses generating these messages are conveyed from one cell to the next by movable protein receptors embedded in the cell walls which rotate like adjustable antennae. These walls are made primarily from fat, their fluidity or hardness determining the movement of the antennae.[4]

3. As for the cells themselves, they are fed by mineral salts and other nutrients which enter the cell at fixed rates. Too much or too little of these nutrients could starve the cells, or poison them, or make them bloated, leading in turn to high blood pressure. Likewise, if any undigested food manages to enter the cell from the blood it will lead to an inflammatory allergic response. It is the fat in the cell walls that prevents this, regulating the flow of minerals, water and food, working in fact like an intelligent filtering mechanism.[5]

4. Oxygen is captured and carried around the body to provide the medium for the reactions of life by haemoglobin, a protein-based transport molecule. However, to move the oxygen across a cell membrane, the body resorts to the ability of the fat substances in the wall to dissolve the oxygen and carry it into the cell.[6]

5. Electricity is generated and conducted in fat cells which work like microscopic capacitors. This is especially important in the myelin sheaths of the nerves, which use electricity to generate their messages.[7]

6. The brain and other vital organs such as eyes and sexual organs are made of highly reactive fat tissue.[8]

Wherever you look in the body, no matter what, you will find fat playing an inseparable role from the body's other nutrients in its metabolic pathways. We shall be looking at these reactions often throughout the book. This idea of fat as part of the body's biochemical unity is one that undermines the notion of fat as the cause of obesity and disease. In fact it's only when we ingest too much fat – and particularly too much of the wrong sorts of fat – that our problems begin, problems that we will also focus on in subsequent chapters. Before that, however, we must find out exactly what fat is.

The fat spine

On average, 95 per cent of all the fat we eat is composed of substances called triglycerides. These are trident-shaped molecules, each 'prong' of which is made from a smaller molecule called a fatty acid. It is these smaller molecules that concern us since they determine the nature of fat, how nutritious it is, how much energy it contains, how it can keep us healthy and, indeed, what sort of threat it might be to our health.

If we break off one of the fatty acid prongs and place it under a powerful microscope, we can see that the prong is a collection of atoms linked together like a chain. Sitting at the centre of this molecule chain is a string of carbon atoms. Mention carbon and one usually thinks of the blackened fragments of charcoal left after a wood fire, inert and lifeless. In fact, together with oxygen, hydrogen and nitrogen, carbon is one of the most essential elements of life, indispensable for its unrivalled stability: it is literally the spine of life.[9] Nearly every chemical reaction in the body that involves the building or demolishing of tissue occurs around this carbon spine. To understand why carbon is so important we have to zoom in even closer to the fatty acid molecule, until it looms around us like a monstrous, city-sized abstract sculpture, and examine the carbon atom.

Carbon, like every atom, carries with it a certain number of electrons, infinitely small satellites that orbit the nucleus. Electrons are seen as particles or waves, changing confusingly from one to the other seemingly at will. However much they elude the attempts of scientists to pin them down, one thing is certain: they are pure energy. This energy generates a powerful electrostatic force that may attract or repel surrounding atoms in the manner of magnetic poles. It is this that enables different atoms to bond together. The number of electrons circling the nucleus determines how many neighbouring atoms it can attach itself to, since each electron can attract only one other atom. Since hydrogen, for example, has only one electron, it is able to bond only with one adjacent atom.

Of the prime elements, carbon carries with it the largest number of electrons and this gives it an enormous advantage. It is able to attract enough atoms of other substances into one place for chemical activity to occur. It is, in effect, biochemical Velcro. This is why carbon sits at the centre of all the important molecular chains in the body – proteins, carbohydrates and fats.

Carbon sits at the centre of the fatty acid molecule in a chain of atoms that can number from 4 to 24. The addition of each extra carbon atom affects the fatty acid's consistency and the overall chemical property of the triglyceride. It is the carbon atom that determines the fatty acid's 'greasiness' and insolubility. The fewer the carbon atoms contained in a fatty acid, the more soluble it will be and the lower its melting point.

Running along this spine of carbon atoms are two lines of hydrogen atoms, one above and one below. Each carbon atom is therefore bonded to two hydrogen atoms in addition to its carbon neighbours on either side. Finally, the chain is topped and tailed by what is called a methyl group at one end (this is where an extra hydrogen atom is substituted for what would be the next carbon atom in the chain; since hydrogen can only make one bond this prevents any more carbon atoms from being added), and an acidic carboxyl at the other (this contains the oxygen in the molecule, making it the 'fuel tank' for any reaction that subsequently takes place).

Although this outlines the basic components of fat, it doesn't begin to illustrate the diversity of substances and functions obtained from this blueprint.

Butter, for example, is composed largely of a fatty acid called butyric acid. Since butyric acid has only four carbon atoms this means that it will dissolve in water fairly easily and have a low melting point in the body of 8°C.[10] Provided you don't eat too much butter, therefore, it will safely be dissolved in the blood, flowing freely around the body until it is burnt as energy. By contrast, stearic acid, a fatty acid found in red meats, has a melting point of 70°C.[11] The higher its melting point, the more likely it is to agglomerate in the

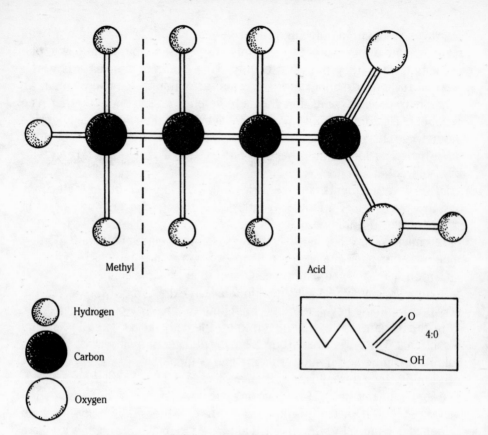

Methyl | | Acid

Hydrogen

Carbon

Oxygen

4:0

Fig 1: A simple fatty acid chain: the spine of four stable carbon atoms surrounded by hydrogen atoms with the methyl group on the left and carboxyl group, or acid, on the right. The fatty acid pictured is butyric acid. Found most commonly in butter, it has the number 4:0 (four carbon atoms and no double bonds). Inset: A stick model shows the molecule's actual shape.

Fig 2: Butyric acid and stearic acid

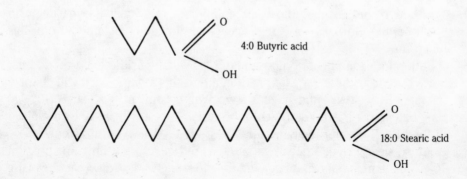

4:0 Butyric acid

18:0 Stearic acid

blood. It will not dissolve, nor flow easily, but form sticky, sludge-like substances that coat the capillary and artery walls of the body, reducing circulation, hardening the vessel walls and raising blood pressure. We'll be examining the implications of this in greater depth in subsequent chapters.

While the length of the carbon chain is one important factor in fat metabolism, another is the question of whether the chain is saturated or unsaturated.

Saturates and unsaturates are two of the great marketing buzz words of our time, employed as often as not to cream off the sales of butter in favour of margarine, full fat in favour of skimmed milk and the truth in favour of public relations gimmickry. The supposed benefit of eating unsaturates, set against the life-threatening consequences of eating saturates, has been used to weave a mythology about fat that has dramatically manipulated public interest and concern. The essence of the message is that polyunsaturates are good for us since they reduce the risks of heart disease, circulatory disorders and obesity, and saturates are bad because they have the opposite effect. While shoppers admit their buying choices are swayed by these concepts, few have any idea what the terms mean. So successful has the campaign been that many people even think that margarine has fewer calories than butter. This is such an interesting and controversial subject that we shall devote the whole of Chapter 7 to it, but in the meantime let us find out what saturates and polyunsaturates are.

Double bonds and the reactions of life

Picture a fatty acid chain, say ten carbon atoms long. Excluding the methyl and carboxyl ends for the moment, this leaves bonding sites for 20 hydrogen atoms, one above and one below each carbon. When each of these bonding sites is occupied – that is, with no space remaining for attracting any more hydrogen atoms – the fatty acid molecule is said to be *saturated*.[12]

Some fatty acids, however, have less than their maximum possible quota of hydrogen atoms. Some are created like this, and a few occur through the removal of one or more pairs of hydrogen atoms by chemical reactions in the body. With less than the full possible number of hydrogen atoms on the molecule, it is said to be *unsaturated*. If the fatty acid has one pair missing, it is *monounsaturated*. More than this makes it *polyunsaturated*. The implications of the removal of the hydrogen on the properties of fatty acids are profound. Let's see why.

Losing two hydrogen atoms leaves two adjacent carbon atoms on the chain, each with one bonding site available. The two will use these extra bonds to join with each other. Since one bond already unites the two of them, this second bonding gives rise to what scientists call 'double bonding'. Double bonding can happen anywhere along the carbon chain. It tends to occur after the third carbon molecule from the methyl end and rarely in a fatty acid with fewer than 16 carbon atoms.

Thanks to its special stability, carbon is vitally important for, and very good at, creating new substances in the body. However, for as long as each of its bonding sites is occupied by hydrogen, the carbon atoms in the fatty acid chain are unable to react. This is why saturated fatty acids are highly inert chemicals. The departure of two or more hydrogen atoms has the effect of removing a screen or plug. While the hydrogen atom was in place occupying all carbon's available bonding sites, carbon was unable to react with the chemicals surrounding the fatty acid. Now, the chemical properties of the carbon atom are exposed to the outside metabolic environment and it is able to facilitate all manner of metabolic activity.

The difference in properties between saturates and unsaturates is remarkable when you consider that they may differ only in respect of two hydrogen atoms. While saturates are chemically inert substances, serving mainly as fuel sources and as insulators, unsaturates, by virtue of their double bonding, are chemically unstable and highly active. The more double bonds on a fatty acid, the more active it becomes. Accordingly, polyunsaturates, those with several double bonds, are highly active, making them vital elements in almost every chemical reaction and physical structure in the body.[13]

Because polyunsaturates tend to perform so many important functions, they are known as *essential fatty acids*. Women's magazines, health cookbooks and margarine and oil manufacturers rhapsodize at length about them. However, nothing is ever as simple as advertisers, marketing and public relations executives would have us believe, especially in the case of nutrition.

Sadly for the ordered world of the food producers' lobby, there are two forms of polyunsaturates. These are called *cis* and *trans*. Each may have the same number of carbon atoms and double bonds as the other but there is one striking difference. Cis is the polyunsaturate form that carries out the billions of life-giving functions in the body. Trans behaves like a subversive double agent, masquerading as the 'good guy' yet all the while undermining the body's health and vitality.[14]

The difference between the two lies in the way that the double bonds are configured. In cis fatty acids with more than one double bond, each gap where the hydrogen atom would be lies on the same side of the carbon chain. As we have seen, every bond between one atom and another needs a free electron to make it happen. Therefore, break a bond by removing one of the atomic partners, hydrogen in the case of a double bond, and the carbon atoms to which it was bonded will be left with a spare electron. If this happens twice in one fatty acid chain there will be two carbon molecules with unpaired electrons. As these electrons are negatively charged they will attempt to repel each other. Therefore, if these exposed double bond sites happen to lie on the same side of the molecule adjacent to each other, the spare electrons, by exerting their repelling force, will cause the entire chain to bend, buckle and kink.

Now imagine that the double bonds are on alternate sides of the chain. They will not kink since, by doing so, unpaired electrons will be brought into close proximity from the opposite sides of the molecule, thereby repelling each other and forcing the chain to unkink. In this case the repelling action keeps the chain perfectly straight. A straight polyunsaturate is called a trans fatty acid. It is highly dangerous because the body can't distinguish between it and its cis equivalent. Therefore, although it is unable to perform any of the functions that the cis form is used for it will still be employed by the body to do so. Trans fatty acids are created mainly inadvertently by a number of food processing methods. This makes it perhaps the world's most widely manufactured and used poison. Read Chapter 2 to discover why.

Fig 3: The cis (kinked) and trans (straight) configurations of a double bond

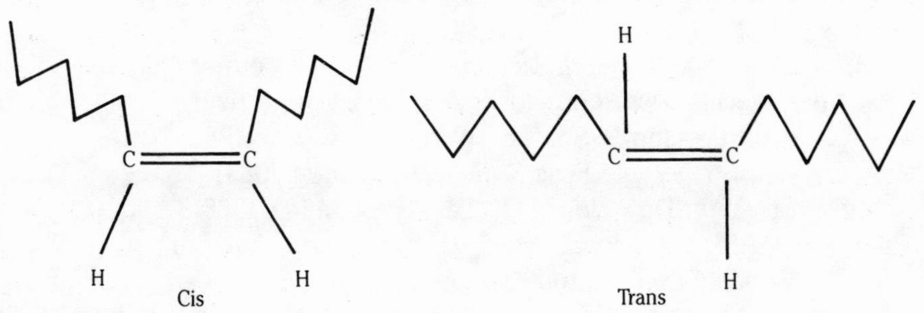

Cis

Trans

References

The literature of fats is burgeoning. However, as you will see from these references at the end of this and each subsequent chapter, not a lot of it is very arresting. There are, however, compelling exceptions, the most notable and readable of which is *Fats and Oils*, by Udo Erasmus, published by Alive Books, of Vancouver, in 1986. This covers comprehensively and comprehendingly all aspects of fat and oil metabolism, processing and marketing, its increasing use in the health supplementation field and the howling misapprehensions the public harbours on the subject. The book was our most inspirational reference source and also directed us to other valuable areas of research in addition to those we already knew about. We mention it at this stage because, as it informed most of the areas we ourselves explored, it seems only right to single out our debt of gratitude at the start.

1 *Life Extension* Pearson D. Shaw S. (Warner: New York 1982)
Mental and Elemental Nutrients Pfeiffer C. (Keats: Connecticut 1975)
Ageless Ageing Kenton L. (Century: London 1985)
2 *The Amino Revolution* Erdmann Dr R. Jones M. (Century: London 1987)
3 *Fats and Oils* Erasmus U. (Alive: Vancouver 1986)
The Chemistry of Life Rose S. (Pelican: London 1985)
4 *The Magic of Magnesium* Trimmer Dr E. (Thorsons: Wellingborough 1987)
Minerals Polunin M. (Thorsons: Wellingborough 1987)
5&6 *The Lively Membranes* Robertson R.N. (Cambridge U. Press: Cambridge 1983)
Structure and Function of the Human Body Memmler R.L. (Lippincott: Philadelphia 1983)
7 *Minerals and Your Health* Mervyn Dr L. (Keats: Connecticut 1981)
8 *Orthomolecular Nutrition* Hoffer A. (Keats: Connecticut 1978)
Life Extension Pearson D. Shaw S. (Warner: New York 1982)
9 *The Chemistry of Life* Rose S. (Pelican: London 1985)
Minerals Erdmann Dr R. Jones M. (Century: London 1988)
10&11 *Lipid Biochemistry* Gurr M. (Chapman and Hall: London 1980)
12 *The Biogenic Diet* Kenton L. (Century: London 1986)
13 'Essential Fatty Acids in Perspective' Sinclair H.M. *Human Nutrition* 38

(1984) 'Trans Fatty Acids – Metabolic and Nutritional Significance' Gurr M. *Nutrition Bulletin* 47 (1986)

14 'Intensification of Essential Fatty Acid Deficiency by Dietary Trans Fatty Acids' Hill E.C. et al. *Journal of Nutrition* 109 (1979)

Chapter 2

Tridents and Trans-Fats

In Chapter 1 we saw how the chemical properties of separate fatty acids vary dramatically, and elicit different effects on the body's metabolism, depending on a few outwardly insignificant factors. These include the number of carbon atoms running along the core of the fatty acid molecule, whether or not this core is saturated with hydrogen atoms or unsaturated with double bonds and indeed whether those unsaturated molecules are cis or trans.

In this and the following chapter, we'll see how the body's metabolic pathways exploit the different fatty acid configurations, forging them into the myriad structures that play such a profound role in the body's vitality and well-being. Fatty acids are the main constituents in literally millions of these structures. By watching as the individual fatty acids are variously incorporated into tissue, and how they lead to the creation of enzymes and hormones, we'll be able to gauge how much influence factors such as cis and trans configurations have on the metabolism. Then, in later chapters, we shall see how this knowledge can be used to practical advantage, helping us to choose which fats and oils to buy, which to stay clear of, and how to use them to maximize their considerable health-giving potential.

We will start with the function for which fat has been most maligned, and for which it is most feared: weight gain.

The fat file

In total, fats and oils account for around 40 per cent of the calories contained in the average daily diet. This works out at around nine calories a gram and is twice as much as either carbohydrate or protein. Rather than an obscure unit of weight measurement, as many people think, a calorie is simply an indication of the molecule's potential energy, or in other words how much heat it would release if it were oxidized. Heat is released from fatty acids by a gradual process of molecular degradation. First the sticky glycerol molecule at the base of the triglyceride trident is broken away, then two carbon atoms at a time are released from the fatty acid chain producing energy and water.[1]

Calories have evolved into the bane of the slimmer's life because only as many calories are released from the food we eat as our bodies need. Since this might be considerably less than the calories contained in food, whatever is left over will be stored. And, since fat is the most efficient medium for storing this caloric energy (as we saw, carrying twice as many calories for the same weight as the alternative food sources), the excess will be converted to fat and stored in adipose tissue beneath the skin. The consequences of such weight gain are well documented: high blood pressure, hardening of the arteries, cardio-vascular disease, a higher incidence rate of cancer, and reduced resistance to illness, to name but a few.

But if more calories are eaten than the body needs for energy, then why does the body not excrete the excess? The answer lies in a mechanism controlled by the thyroid gland called the basal metabolism rate. This apportions the body's food supplies rather as a grudging quartermaster distributes equipment in a forces barracks. It supplies the body with enough energy to meet its needs in times of plenty but is much more abstemious in times of famine. Such a tendency harks back to prehistory when our ancestors foraged and hunted for food. They would often have to go hungry for long periods, making strict internal rationing a practical necessity.[2]

Nowadays, particularly in the West where food mountains have become part of the landscape, there is very little likelihood of going without food. Nonetheless, when we eat more than we strictly need, the body will still jealously conserve it for times of famine even though we know they will not arise. This is nowhere more true than in the case of carbohydrate. Even though it is the energy source preferred by the body, if consumed in excess, it will still be turned to fat. Carbohydrates, or starches, are complex molecules created from the bonding of simpler sugar molecules such as sucrose, glucose and fructose. The complex forms are broken apart into their individual sugar constituents by enzymes and this allows the sugars to be oxidized to produce energy, splitting away pairs of carbon atoms in the same way as fat.

Ideally, carbohydrate intake should not exceed the body's energy require-ments – that is, all the available sugar should be burnt by physical activity.

However, as man has become a largely sedentary creature, a certain buildup of carbohydrate is almost inevitable. Even then, though, nature provides carbohydrate with certain important chemical co-factors such as B vitamins, fibre and minerals to ensure that the buildup is not dangerous. These co-factors slow down digestion and provide the body with materials to help the enzymes fully metabolize the sugars that have been consumed. In effect, they make the thyroid quartermaster a little more generous with the food it releases to be burnt as energy, and this ensures that most of the sugar is burnt at the rate at which it is absorbed. [3]

The foods containing these co-factors are called complex carbohydrates. However, thanks to modern industrial food processing producing sources of refined carbohydrates, such as white bread, pasta, pre-prepared sauces, cakes and biscuits, much of the carbohydrate we eat today has had its co-factors stripped away. This is absorbed much more quickly and – in the absence of the co-factors necessary for helping to metabolize it – quickly builds up in the body to be converted to long-chain saturated fatty acids. [4] These carbohydrates are called 'empty calories' since they provide a lavish source of energy with no means for the body to take advantage of it. [5]

Since saturated fats will agglomerate harmfully in the body, it's important to understand why they work in this way. So let's take a closer look.

Saturates synopsis

Saturated fatty acids contain anything from 4 to 24 carbon atoms. Since each available bond on each carbon atom is saturated – that is, fully occupied by hydrogen atoms – such fat is unable to attract electrons from atoms in other molecules. This makes bonding with other substances very difficult and saturates are therefore extremely slow to react to, or cause, chemical activity. Similarly, the longer the carbon chain, the higher its melting point.

Saturated fatty acids with up to 10 carbon atoms – such as capric acid which is found in goats' milk – are liquid at body temperature (37°C) but below this they become increasingly sticky. Stearic acid, the chain containing 18 carbon molecules, named after the Greek word for fat and found in especially high amounts in beef, pork and mutton, has a melting point of 70°C (about 160°F). The higher the melting point, the more likely these fatty acids are to form sticky clots in cells, organs and arteries. This is compounded by the tendency of these straight, flat molecules to agglomerate one on top of the other. Remember, of all the fatty acids, it's only the cis-configured unsaturates that are kinked and therefore unable to stack closely together. [6]

Some saturates are actually a useful, if hardly necessary, fuel source. Saturated fatty acids with a spine of fewer than 14 carbon atoms are usually burnt to release energy and heat for the body (measured in calories). Those with carbon atoms numbering between 16 and 18 can be utilized as energy sources if the body is running short of its normal fuel supplies such as carbohydrate. Alternatively, they may be stored as fat for insulation and cushioning purposes.

In general, provided you don't eat too much fat, there is no reason why saturated fats should harm you. For example, since butyric acid, the fat found in butter, is fluid at body temperature, small amounts will not endanger the arteries by threatening to clog them up. It is also an excellent source of energy. However, if we eat more butter than we strictly need for energy purposes, the thyroid quartermaster will store this away to guard against future famine. With its short carbon chain making it very fluid and easily soluble in water, butyric acid itself is very hard to store. The body prefers something more inert and stable that can be stored with a minimum of fuss. Therefore, the body converts it into something more easily manageable, namely a fatty acid with 16 carbon atoms in its chain. This fatty acid is much more sticky and has a melting point high above our body temperature. Too much butter, therefore, will start to clog up the arteries and lead to excess body fat. [7]

It is impossible to say how much fat it is safe to eat since it varies from person to person depending on indeterminate factors such as age, size, weight, the amount of regular physical activity, and metabolic rate (the genetically determined speed with which growth and regeneration is carried out). This, of course, tends to undermine the value of a so-called calorie controlled diet, as each person's requirements are different.

Bearing these facts in mind it's easy to wonder whether long-chain saturated fatty acids are of any use to the body at all. They seem to clog the body up with their heavy, cumbersome, unmoving and inert consistency, like syrup injected into a finely honed clockwork movement. At best, they supply the body with fuel that can be derived from other sources much more practicably. In fact, despite all this, saturated fatty acids are vital. Their relative stability is necessary for providing structural support to the cell membrane. They also regulate the chemical activity of their unsaturated counterparts by shielding them from undesired reactions. Furthermore, they protect the body's vital organs from the pounding and shock of everyday life – and simply walking along a pavement sends severe shock waves through the body – by cushioning them in a deep, protective sheath.[8] Before we see how they achieve these feats, let's look at their unsaturated counterparts.

Polyunsaturated précis

Polyunsaturates are rarely shorter than 16 carbon molecules long, although monounsaturates, those fatty acids with only one double bond, may contain as few as 10 carbon atoms.

In order to distinguish the different types of fatty acids, and in particular unsaturates, scientists have developed a number of methods of classification. The most comprehensible means of expressing the chemical properties of these chemicals is by a method which describes the configuration of the carbon spine numerically. The numbers in these formulae equate respectively to the overall number of carbon atoms in the chain, the number of double bonds and the position of these bonds on the carbon spine. For example:

As shown in Fig 4, palmiroleic acid has 16 carbon atoms and 1 double bond which, counting from the methyl end, occurs on the spine's seventh atom. Hence 16: 1n-7.

Since oleic acid has 18 carbon molecules and 1 double bond which occurs on the ninth carbon atom from the methyl end, it is represented as 18: 1n-9.

Fig 4: Palmitoleic Acid

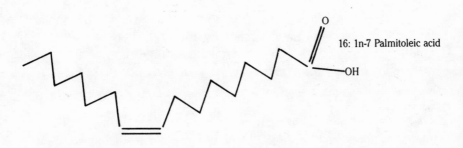

16: 1n-7 Palmitoleic acid

Fig 5: Oleic Acid

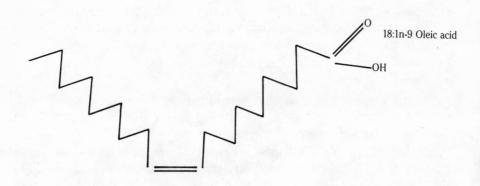

18:1n-9 Oleic acid

The number corresponding to the double bond's position in the molecule, in this case 9, has a particularly important bearing on the recognition of fatty acids. This is called the *omega number* and oleic acid thus belongs to the omega 9 group of fatty acids.

Although monounsaturates do have a certain nutritional value to the body, the fatty acids that are most important for your health are the polyunsaturates belonging to the omega 6 and 3 series. These two groups are headed respectively by linoleic acid (omega 6) and linolenic acid (omega 3), both names deriving from linum, the Latin word for flax (this is why the oil obtained from flax is usually called linseed oil). Linoleic acid, an 18-strong carbon molecule, has two double bonds, the first starting at the sixth carbon atom and is therefore described as: 18: 2n-6. Linolenic acid also has an 18-strong carbon spine but has three double bonds, the first of which appears on the third carbon atom: 18: 3n-3.

Both these fatty acids are of vital importance to the body's metabolism and since they cannot be manufactured by the body they are called *dietary essential* fatty acids.[9] The other important unsaturated fatty acids can be made by the body itself. With proper enzymes your body can make them from the others and although they are necessary for health they are not called dietary essentials.

Recently, the dietary essential fatty acids have been the subject of considerable medical research. In 1982, the Nobel prize for medicine was awarded to

Professor J.R. Vane for his work into the way omega 3 prevented heart disease. [10]

But the importance of these substances was first realized as far back as 1929 when omega 6 was found to promote thin blood and high energy levels.

This work was extended in a famous piece of work carried out by Dr H.O. Bang in the clinical chemistry department of the University of Alborge, Denmark, when he examined the health of a large group of Eskimos leading a traditional lifestyle, whose largely all-meat diet was high in cholesterol from whale and seal blubber. Of the 2400 Eskimos in the group, only three showed any sign of heart disease and none had diabetes, figures which, considering their diets, seemed to fly in the face of accepted medical wisdom. However, when they were moved from their own natural diets to an ordinary Danish equivalent, the rates of cardio-vascular disease increased astronomically. It was then that the link was made between the high quantities of omega 3 obtained from the diet of fresh fish and the Eskimos' almost supernatural levels of health. [11]

Subsequent research showed that omega 6 and 3 essential fatty acids play a significant role in regulating the levels of saturated fatty acids. [12] By working as the reactive components of special carrier molecules called plasma lipo-proteins, they prevent blood platelets from becoming sticky and agglutinating, and reduce the levels of plasma cholesterol. More important still, they play major roles in the cell walls. Due to their double bonds they possess negative electrical charges. This turns them into conduits, conducting electrons and energy through the cell molecule. In this way, nerve messages can be carried from cell to cell and the energy needed to power the metabolic reactions of life supplied wherever it is needed. It also means that the electrical impulses from the brain, constantly criss-crossing the entire body, are properly directed and kept apart like express trains crossing each other's tracks at a large junction. If these impulses were to cross inadvertently, due to a deficiency of the essential fatty acids, they would create a short circuit and lead to neurological problems such as schizophrenia. [13]

Linoleic acid (LA) deficiency has been linked to eczema and psoriasis, hair loss, glandular atrophy – leading in turn to infertility, growth deficiency and weight disorders – water loss, reduced immune function, behavioural difficulties, poor healing, miscarriages and circulatory disorders. Likewise, lino-lenic acid (LNA) deficiency is also thought to play a part in growth retardation and abnormal behavioural changes as well as muscle weakness, impairment of vision, impaired learning abilities, the spread of rheumatic and arthritic disorders, and deteriorating motor co-ordination. [14]

Since longer and longer unsaturated chains can be created from these two substances, they are the parent molecules of a family of so-called omega 6 and omega 3 fatty acids. As the number of double bonds on an unsaturate is the primary measure of its chemical potential, increasing the number of double bonds increases the molecule's metabolic reactivity.

The greater number of unpaired electrons, for example, gives the fatty acid the ability not only to direct but to generate electrical currents. This is vital in an organ such as the brain where a cross-currenting network of messages are sparking through the organ at incredible speeds. The brain is a complex reference library and before any message can be relayed to the appropriate part of the body in response to a stimulus – such as ordering the mouth to salivate when the smell of cooked food is sensed – a series of relays inside the brain flash from one source of stored information to another searching for precedents to these actions and corroboration before approving the impulse. Billions of messages are passing through like this every minute. Imagine one single telephone exchange for the whole world and it gives some notion of the complexity. If the messages are not conveyed quickly enough, or if approval for actions is given when it shouldn't have been, behavioural and mechanical difficulties will arise. The brain therefore needs a medium that will carry these messages quickly and efficiently and, thanks to the electrical potential of the polyunsaturates, it uses essential fatty acids to solve its communications problems.[15]

Polyunsaturates also attract oxygen. Reacting with the fatty acids, this oxygen produces a series of metabolic pathways that result in the creation of prostaglandins, a series of control chemicals that determine all manner of activity including hormone production and control, immune response and maintaining healthy skin. These will be discussed further in Chapter 3.

Essential fatty acids are vital for the health and function of the body but they cannot accomplish their assigned biochemical tasks alone. For this they need the triple-fatty-acid molecules, the triglycerides and the phosphatides.

Triglyceride terminology

As we've seen, fat is more than merely a way of storing excess body fuel. Saturates, because of their stability and inert qualities, make excellent insulators, protecting the body against extremes of heat and cold as well as acting as the 'safety belts' of the vital organs. Essential fatty acids (omega 3 and 6 polyunsaturates), on the other hand, because of their high level of potential chemical reactivity, are used in large proportions in cell membranes and for functions that demand intense biochemical activity. Such functions include roles in the sense organs, testes, ovaries, adrenal glands, and brain cells.[16]

However, fats are used for a great many more separate tasks than there are differing configurations of fatty acids to perform them. This is why triglycerides – the trident-like fat molecules – are so important. Of all the fat we eat, 95 per cent is one form or another of triglyceride. Using its glycerol molecule as the sticky base to bind the separate fatty acids, the triglyceride can gather together three chains in many different combinations. Bearing in mind that saturated fatty acids have links of carbon atoms numbering from 4 to 24 and that unsaturated fatty acids can be made even longer into superunsaturates should the need arise, the number of potential combinations is huge. Accordingly, fatty acids are rarely used singly but rather in these triple combinations.

While all triglycerides are not the same, over three-quarters contain one or more of either palmitic, stearic or oleic acids with reserves of other fats such as LA and LNA. Whether a substance is fat or oil depends on the amount of a particular fatty acid – saturated, mono- or polyunsaturated – contained in the triglyceride. Animal fat, for instance, is composed largely of triglycerides that have almost no essential fatty acids at all so it is inert and melts from a fat to an oil only at a temperature way above that of the body. Flax and safflower oil, on the other hand, have little but essential fatty acids and will not solidify from their oil state to a fat until very low temperatures have been attained. The body therefore must break these foreign triglycerides down before obtaining the fatty acids which it needs from them.

Phosphatide facts

Along with the triglycerides, there is another, smaller, but no less important group of lipids called phosphatides.[17] The difference between the two is that whereas triglycerides hold three fatty acids in the glycerol base, one of the three prongs of a phosphatide is phosphate molecule. This is a crucial difference. The role of the triglycerides is essentially to act as insulators and protectors, agglomerating in large clumps in the water-based environment of the body. The charged polarity of the phosphate, on the other hand, enables the phosphate to repel from, and disperse over, water to form wafer-thin membranes. This produces the skin not only of every cell but of every organelle within the cell such as the energy-producing mitochondria.

Like triglycerides, phosphatides exploit the conflicting properties of different fatty acids to build the cell membrane. A certain amount of rigidity in the cell wall is necessary for ensuring that the receptor points receive and distribute the correct nerve messages, enzymes and hormones. At the same time, a degree of fluidity is important so that the cell retains a certain amount of lateral and transverse movement. On a macro scale this means that skin, muscles and organs retain a degree of flexibility and softness, while microscopically it allows for satisfactory diffusion of mineral atoms and lets through the roving protein molecules which routinely transport other food molecules through the wall.

The balance between rigidity and fluidity is maintained thanks to the phosphatide in the cell wall carrying a saturated fatty acid with a long carbon chain in the outer prong and an unsaturated fatty acid in the middle. The saturates, since they are inert, straight-chained molecules, will stack together very tightly and insulate the highly reactive essential fatty acids from causing each other to spark into activity. The cis-kinked polyunsaturate, on the other hand, will prevent the molecules from stacking too tightly while the polarized phosphate molecule will cause them to form spontaneously into two thin layers of fat, lining up top to tail like fluid brickwork.

This combination of closely-stacked saturate with the kinked, unstable unsaturate creates a strong, stable cell wall which is nonetheless flexible almost to the point of fluidity. The ratio of saturate to unsaturate differs depending on where the molecule is situated in the body. The more sensitive and prone to chemical reaction the cell or hormone is, the greater the need for unsaturates to be included in the phosphatide trident: brain cells and the cells found in glands such as the testes, adrenal and thymus have the most highly polyunsaturated fatty acids in their structures.

Phosphatides are also used to maintain the integrity of the cell wall by determining which substances are allowed in. A deficiency of the omega 6 and 3 fatty acids will cause the body to substitute fewer unsaturated molecules in the contributing phosphatide. This may lead to a loss of impermeability, allowing in improperly digested proteins, bacteria and viruses, as well as the possibility of carcinogens. It's not surprising, therefore, that omega 6 and 3 deficiency is being linked to an increasingly broad cross-section of illnesses including poor mental development, poor vision, dry, scaly skin and inflam-mation such as that associated with rheumatic diseases.

Which brings us more or less full circle back to those bionutritional imposters, the trans-configured polyunsaturates. As we've seen, essential fatty acids such as LA and LNA perform a variety of basic and crucial functions in the body. They accomplish these thanks to two main characteristics: double bonding and a kinked configuration. Trans fatty acids, while possessing the same number of double bonds, are not kinked. This is a feature that the body is unable to distinguish. These unkinked molecules compete with their cis counterparts, and are therefore incorporated into the vast diversity of chemical structures without possessing the necessary reactive properties to perform the functions for which they have been designated. Not only will they stack closely in a manner resembling the saturates, but the fact that their double bonds are on opposing sides of the molecule means that they will only partially link up with the enzymes and hormones that help to facilitate these chemical reactions.[18]

Imagine the damage if these chemicals replaced the kinked essential fatty acids in the brain.[19] The behavioural difficulties that may result from the brain messages being poorly transmitted may lead to depression, anxiety and even more profound forms of mental abnormality, not to mention motor disorders such as lack of physical co-ordination.[20] Equally, there will be a loss of skin pliability, a reduced immune function and less food and oxygen distributed inside the cells.

Trans fatty acids are almost unknown in nature. They occur only when the triumphant technological wizardry of modern food processing techniques is unleashed on the essential fatty acids, particularly when enormous physical pressures and temperatures are brought to bear on oil sources to extract their contents and when oils are transformed into margarines. For more on this subject, turn to Chapters 5, 6 and 7. As for Chapter 3 it's time we met a few of fat's close relations.

References

1,6,9,13,14&18 *Fats and Oils* Erasmus U. (Alive: Vancouver 1986)

2 *Psychodietetics* Cheraskin E. (Bantam: New York 1978)

3&5 *Life Extension* Pearson D. Shaw S. (Warner: New York 1982)

4 'Serum Cholesterol Response to Dietary Cholesterol' Hegsted D. *Am. J. Clinical Nutrition* 44 (1986)

5 *Biogenic Diet* Kenton L. (Century: London 1986)

7 'Relationship of diet to the fatty acid composition of human adipose tissue structure and stored lipids' Field C. et al. *Am. J. Clinical Nutrition* 42 (1985)

8 *Mental and Elemental Nutrients* Pfeiffer C. (Keats: Connecticut 1975)

9 'Essential fatty acids in perspective' Sinclair H.M. *Human Nutrition* 38 (1984) *Essential Fatty Acids* Sinclair H.M. (Butterworths: London 1958) *Fatty Acids* Pryde E.H. (Am. Oil Chemists Society: Champaign, Illinois) *Physiological Chemistry of Lipids in Mammals* Masoro E.J. (Saunders: Philadelphia 1968)

10 'Prostaglandins and the cardio-vascular system' Vane J.R. *British Heart Journal* (1983)

11 'The Composition of Food Consumed by Greenland Eskimos' *Acta Medica Scandinavia* 200 (1976)
'Plasma Lipids in Greenland Eskimos' *Acta Medica Scandinavia* 192 (1972)

12 'Low prevalence of coronary heart disease, psoriasis, asthma and rheumatoid arthritis in Eskimos' Horrobin D. (Efamol Research Institute, Kentville, Nova Scotia, Canada) *Medical Hypotheses* 22 (1987)

15 *Orthomolecular Psychiatry* Hawkins D. Pauling L. (eds) (Freeman: San Francisco 1973) 'A case of human linoleic acid deficiency involving neurological abnormalities' *Am. J. Clinical Nutrition* 35 (1982)

16 'Nutritional Properties of Triglycerides and Saturated Fatty Acids of Medium Chain Length' Kaunitz H. et al. *J. Am. Oil. Chemists Society* 35 (1958)

17 *Life Extension* Pearson D. Shaw S. (Warner: New York 1982)

19 *Ageless Ageing* Kenton L. (Century: London 1985)

20 'Intensification of Essential Fatty Acid Deficiency by Dietary Trans Fatty Acids' Hill E.C. et al. *J. Nutrition* 109 (1979)

Chapter 3

Fat Relatives

Simply eating food containing the fats our bodies need for a healthy metabolism is only the first stage of the process that will eventually see them incorporated as components of hormones and tissue. Before they can go any further, the individual essential fatty acids, monounsaturates and saturates have to be removed from the larger food molecules. This means having to disassemble those molecules, dismantling them bit by bit, rather like a building firm might demolish an old house to obtain the bricks which it will use as building materials for a new one. [1]

Comprehensively dismantling the molecules in this way is a crucial element of nutrient assimilation. Absorbing the large food molecules through the gut intact is impractical for several reasons. For one, the form of these molecules, constructed as they are in complex configurations, is of little use to the body. It has its own highly individualized needs which can only be met by the molecule's components. In the same way, a new house wouldn't be built from existing gable ends and chimney stacks, but from scratch – the bricks that formerly made up those features now constituting completely new ones. The second reason for taking the molecules apart is that any complex tissue originating from a foreign organism is treated by the body as an invader and it generates a legion of white blood cells and macrophages to dissolve it. [2] Clearly, dietary fat must be broken down comprehensively into simple fatty acid molecules before it can be absorbed through the gut wall – or mucosa – and filtered into the bloodstream. [3]

The first stage of fat digestion occurs in the stomach where lipase enzyme tears it away from other types of food. After this it moves into the small intestine where it is mixed with more lipase enzymes from the pancreas and bile from the gall bladder. Bile has a detergent effect, increasing the fat's surface area by emulsifying it into a stream of droplets. This is immensely important since fat molecules tend to stick together in large indigestible clumps. These clumps are broken down by the bile, and as the fat passes through the duodenum, it is attacked by the lipase enzymes secreted by the pancreas. Enzymes are protein-based substances and there is a different sort for each category of fat. They break open the triglycerides and phosphatides, tearing away the fatty acid and phosphate chains from the glycerol bases.[4]

The liberated fatty acids are then collected by a separate set of lipoprotein molecules called *chylomicrons* and transported individually across the mucosa.[5] Once through the mucosal barrier they are distributed by a complex intracellular carrier network via the liver to the cells. The substances they encounter on this journey from stomach to tissue and the way in which these substances influence fat metabolism is what we shall look at in this chapter. Our first encounter on this metabolic odyssey is with one whose name is enough to chill the more assiduously weight-conscious reader's blood – cholesterol!

Cholesterol – cellular anti-hero

As with many naturally-occurring substances maligned by science, cholesterol has had a bad press. A hard, waxy chemical, it is associated with various forms of cardio-vascular disease including high blood pressure, angina, hardening of the arteries and stroke. Fears of the effects of cholesterol on the circulatory system first surfaced in 1913 when a group of white rabbits had the misfortune to be fed on a high-cholesterol diet by a Russian pathologist called Nikolai Anichkov.[6] The diet caused a discernible hardening of the rabbits' arteries and clearly suggested a correlation between atherosclerosis and cholesterol. Ever since, it has been regarded as a dietary bane with each new study uncovering fresh evidence of the menacing ramifications of cholesterol in the diet.

One or two facts, though, call this view into question: the incidence rate of cardio-vascular disease has grown enormously since Anichkov fattened up his rabbits, yet cholesterol consumption has remained relatively stable. Further-more, cholesterol is an important regulating component that protects against exhaustion and collapse.[7] Using cholesterol, the body produces a series of stress-combat hormones and mediates the health and efficiency of the cell membranes. It is found in the nerve fibre sheaths, white matter of the brain and adrenal glands.[8] It also helps to regulate the body's salt and water balance. It is regarded by the body as such an important metabolic aid that every cell has a mechanism to manufacture its own supply. Up to two grams are produced internally every day, four times the amount found in our diets. This renders the idea of dietary cholesterol as the cause of cardio-vascular problems partly redundant, although the fact that many of the co-factors necessary for helping the body to metabolize cholesterol are refined out of the food is an important one. To look for the causes of cardio-vascular disease we obviously have to dig a little deeper.[9]

Cholesterol – origins and uses

As with most products of metabolic pathways, oxidation starts the synthesis of cholesterol. In Chapter 2 we saw how fatty acids produce energy when pairs of carbon atoms (acetate groups) are removed from the chain by the oxidative process. This occurs to some extent not only with fats but with sugars – the body's main source of energy – and, in extreme cases of starvation, protein. To create cholesterol, the body links these pairs of newly liberated carbon atoms together, snips a few away, and arrives at a cholesterol molecule 27 carbon atoms in length. With so many carbon atoms in each molecule its hard, waxy consistency comes as no surprise, nor does its melting point of 149°C.[10]

In terms of its work in the body, we first meet cholesterol in the small intestine since it is the main component of bile, the acid used to emulsify our dietary fat. The cholesterol used for this purpose is made in the liver which is the single largest source of the substance. The liver regulates the amount of cholesterol in the body, determining not only how much bile acid is produced but also the amount of bile and cholesterol stored in the gall bladder and later to be excreted into the intestine.[11]

Our next encounter with cholesterol is at the cell membrane where it has an important part to play in sustaining the membrane's health and integrity against invasion from foreign substances. As we have seen the membranes are kept in a state of 'structured fluidity' by the balancing actions of the different fatty acids in the triglycerides and the phosphatides. The rigidity given the cell wall by the inert, closely stacking saturated fatty acids is balanced by the instability of the cis-linked polyunsaturate and vice versa. As with most mechanisms in the body, however, this ideal equilibrium is subjected to continual disruptive change.[12] The passage of different foods across the membrane, and the need for the protein receptors embedded in the wall to move in order to relay and receive their hormonal messages, mean that the cell wall is in a state of becoming alternatively more and less fluid than the norm.

Other, less desirable, factors also cause changes in the cell wall. Alcohol, for example, dissolves a certain amount of the saturated fatty acids so that, in losing its structure, the wall becomes progressively more fluid. When this happens in the nervous system, the messages transmitted by the protein receptors of neighbouring cells grow increasingly uncoordinated and we experience this as the classic symptoms of drunkenness – slurred speech, vertiginous dizziness and mild hallucinations. [13]

The body simply cannot afford to let this progress too far in the cell. If the cell wall becomes too fluid it might fall apart. It therefore injects cholesterol into the wall to increase its stability and stave off any serious problems. As the alcohol effects wear off, the cholesterol is slowly withdrawn. (One of the causes of alcoholism is the fact that so much cholesterol has to be pumped into the cell wall that it becomes permanently hardened. Simply to keep the cell wall fluid and stay sober, therefore, an alcoholic must drink excessively; to become drunk he or she must progressively increase the alcohol intake.) Of course, cholesterol isn't used only for alcohol. It is needed to a greater or lesser extent all the time. Maintaining the integrity of the cell wall ensures that food is passed into the cell and that skin tissue is well oiled. [14]

Continuing on our journey around the body, we will also meet cholesterol in the glands as it is the derivative of a number of steroid hormones. These include the female sex hormones, oestrogen and progesterone, and the male hormone, testosterone. Similarly, it is a component of the adrenal cortico-steroids – mineralocorticoid and glucocorticoid – the substances which help the body to prepare for its fight or flight stress responses by manufacturing glucose in anticipation of greater energy needs. Therefore, stress is a great stimulant for producing cholesterol. [15]

Cholesterol is also the parent molecule of a metabolic pathway that creates a hormone called aldosterone. This works with the kidneys to regulate the body's water balance, retaining or excreting sodium from the renal tubes depending on the body's needs at the time. A cholesterol deficiency is likely to lead to abnormal water retention; in turn, this can lead to high blood pressure. [16]

Most people would be surprised to find that a lack of cholesterol is linked to high blood pressure since the reverse is usually thought to hold true. So why is cholesterol linked so firmly with cardio-vascular disease? One theory has it that it is cholesterol's tendency to repair damaged tissue that proves to be its undoing. To understand why this is so means entering the world of an imperceptibly small, but potentially highly dangerous, particle called a free radical.

Cholesterol – the radical departure

The colourful name amply evokes a picture of the damage and destruction that free radicals may cause. They are linked with disease, debilitation, degeneration and accelerated ageing. In essence, they are molecules, one of whose atoms has an unpaired electron.[17] In Chapter 1 we saw how the electrons of each atom act as molecular cement, attracting and bonding carbon, hydrogen and oxygen atoms together to create fatty acids. We also saw that with the departure of a pair of hydrogen atoms the vacated electron sites of the two neighbouring carbon atoms create a double bond. In nature, everything is ordered in this way so that any electron freed by a chemical reaction will link with another atom. At least, it is usually.

However, every now and then, during the process of energy production caused by oxidation, one electron rotates itself free of its atom and spins off into oblivion without automatically having another electron to replace it. This leaves an unpaired electron. Naturally, this electron will then seek to bond itself with another and in order to achieve this will literally scavenge the nearest available electron it can find. In doing so it robs another molecule of an electron and this in turn sets out to find a replacement elsewhere. If unchecked, this 'free radicalism' will spread through the tissue like a biochemical earth tremor.[18]

The effect of this activity on the protein structures of the body such as arterial linings is similar to the effects of subsidence on part of a brick wall: while part of the wall remains where it was, the other part has shifted slightly, tearing a crack where the two planes meet. Normally, free radical activity is limited by specially created enzymes. However, when these enzymes are limited by common dietary deficiencies, or when there is an increase in poisons such as carbon monoxide or heavy metals such as lead and aluminium, free radical activity commences with a vengeance.[19]

Such activity will lead to ruptures in the cell membranes and, in turn, of the reticulated protein structure of the arterial lining. Bringing to bear all the defensive resources it can, the body attempts to bridge these fissures with the substance it uses to effect repairs and control cell fluidity – cholesterol. If the damage is great enough, so much cholesterol will be introduced that it may become a health hazard by combining the calcium and phosphorus circulating in the blood and further hardening the artery or tissue walls. This cholesterol will also increase the stickiness of the blood platelets, reducing circulation and leading in turn to the possibility of high blood pressure, stroke, deafness, blindness, heart attack, and heart and kidney failure. [20] Discovering cholesterol in such large quantities – standing, as it were, over the corpse with a loaded gun – it is easy to understand why it is blamed for so many of the problems associated with cardio-vascular disease.

One method does exist for doctors to predict the rise in cholesterol build up before it happens and this involves measuring the concentration in the blood of a group of substances called plasma lipoproteins. These are chemicals that operate like high-speed couriers, sheathing the cholesterol, and sundry forms of fat, in a membraneous sac of phosphatides and protein then carrying them to the tissue as needed. These chemicals fall into two main categories – high density lipoproteins (HDL) and low density lipoproteins (LDL). [21] LDLs carry cholesterol from the mucosa to the liver and then on for distribution to the individual cells. HDLs conduct cholesterol on the return journey, hauling it back to the liver where it is converted to bile acid and excreted into the stools.

Although overall cholesterol content and its concomitant risk of cardio-vascular disease is often judged by adding together the amounts in the blood of these two lipoproteins, this method can distort and disguise the true picture. If, for example, the total measurement appeared low, the obvious conclusion would be that cholesterol levels were healthy and unlikely to build up to cardio-vascular-disease-threatening levels in the near future. However, until the ratio of HDL to LDL was examined it would be impossible to know if this were true. It may be, for example, that the percentage of HDL ferrying cholesterol away from the cells was very low, therefore establishing that a high percentage of the total consisted of LDL moving the cholesterol into the cells. [22] No matter how low the overall lipoprotein level, therefore, this would indicate that cholesterol was building up in the cells faster than it was being removed.

The natural ratio of HDL to LDL is 3:5 [23] and discerning variances from this mean is considered to be the only accurate way of predicting an increase in cholesterol. Of course, with an adequate nutritional profile, cholesterol is not likely to become excessive in the first place. One of the best ways of ensuring that cholesterol is metabolized effectively is to keep your diet serviced with adequate levels of the next fat-related substance we are to meet – lecithin.

Lecithin

Lecithin is a phosphatide high in essential fatty acids. It has a close working relationship with cholesterol and is the parent molecule of a substance called choline. The highest quality lecithin is found in soya bean oil where 57 per cent of its contents are linoleic acid (LA) and 9 per cent linolenic acid (LNA).[24] Choline is important for helping cholesterol and other saturated fats to move around the body. Since these are essentially inert chemicals, at best reluctantly participating in chemical reactions, otherwise working simply by preventing them from occurring, they need a strong biochemical impetus with which to mobilize them. By helping provide that impetus, choline is part of what scientists call the 'lipotrophic factor'.[25]

Were it not for the lipotrophic factor, saturates and cholesterol would veer towards a state of permanent agglomeration, building up in the liver, heart and arteries. Very simply, choline works by emulsifying these molecules, keeping the cholesterol soluble so that the plasma lipoproteins can transport it around the body more efficiently. This also helps to detoxify and prevent a buildup of fat in the liver.

Another important role for choline occurs when three molecules join together to form a super-active molecule called phosphatidyl choline.[26] This reacts in turn with vitamin B5 to create a neurotransmitter called acetyl-choline. Neurotransmitters are a series of chemicals whose responsibilities include relaying messages from the brain, through the nerve cells and into the body at large. Acetylcholine conveys messages that dictate several different categories of response including co-ordinating muscle control, giving tone to gut muscles, calming mental and physical arousal after stress, and aiding memory. Nutritionists sometimes suggest that victims of insomnia and nocturnal restlessness, both of which may be symptoms of choline shortage, take a supplement of lecithin before bed.

The word 'lecithin' is derived from the Greek for egg yolk, since this food is one of its most concentrated sources. Herein lies an interesting lesson. When talking about the harm that an individual food such as cholesterol can cause us, we tend to forget that nature has evolved an intricate, and comprehensive, network of regulators and balancers. Therefore, the fact that eggs contain cholesterol – a fact that many commentators have focused upon to recommend that we eat fewer eggs – is more than compensated for by the regulatory properties of the lecithin. Most substances only become a menace when the food in which they are found has its balancing co-factors refined away in the name of convenience or cosmetic appearance.[27]

In the light of this, it should come as no surprise to find that producers are developing certain foods with strains of fatty acid containing as little as 3 per cent LNA instead of the optimal 9 per cent found in peanut and soya bean oils. This in turn means that the quality of lecithin in the food is considerably reduced.[28] Meat and dairy products resulting from intensive farming methods increasingly contain lecithin with oleic acid (DA 18: 1n-9) substituted for most of the LNA. This, of course, helps to increase the food's shelf life by reducing the lecithin's chemical potential to attract oxygen. The fact that it also reduces its ability to dissolve gallstones, emulsify fat and prevent cholesterol deposition in the arterial linings, not to mention promote a healthily functioning brain, is an irrelevance to the retail barons.

Lecithin has one other role, too: in the thymus gland as a precursor of the prostaglandins. In order to see just how important these fat-derived substances are to your metabolism, let's find out what they do.

Prostaglandins – the mayfly metabolites

The reactive lifespan of a prostaglandin is over practically as soon as it begins. Any one of the 30 or so yet identified is brought into existence via a complicated metabolic pathway, issues a single command to a specific part of the body, and, in doing so, destroys itself, disappearing back into the metabolic vortex to be remetabolized elsewhere. But in that brief moment of reactive potential, the orders it issues affect the entire body. Prostaglandins make capillaries dilate, release armies of immune-response cells to repel the invasion of viruses and bacteria, trigger inflammatory responses to allergens and help regulate calcium metabolism, to name only a few of their roles.[29]

Prostaglandins (PG) are created from the omega 6 and omega 3 essential fatty acids, LA and LNA. So named because they were first discovered in the prostate gland, there are three families of prostaglandin: PGE1, PGE2 and PGE3. These are produced from metabolic pathways which see enzymes inserting double bonds into LA and LNA to create increasingly unstable and chemically reactive molecules. PGE1 and PGE2 come into being as a result of chemical action on linoleic acid (18: 2n-6). This is turned progressively into gamma linolenic acid

(GLA 18: 3n-6), dihomogamma linolenic acid (DGLA 20: 3n-6) and arachidonic acid (20: 4n-6).

PGE1, which is created by DGLA, is perhaps the best known of the prostaglandins since its effects, primarily on the circulatory system, are profound and numerous. It protects the body against the consequences of excessive plasma cholesterol by preventing blood platelets from sticking together, slows down cholesterol production in the liver and makes the capillaries dilate to reduce the chance of blood clots and to keep blood pressure down. It also contributes to a reduction in blood pressure by acting as a diuretic, ordering the kidneys to remove some of the water circulating in the plasma and cells. Women suffering from the bloated sensations symptomatic of their menstrual periods often find relief by taking supplements high in PGE1, but more on that later. PGE1 also helps the body to utilize insulin – the glucose-regulating hormone – more efficiently so that energy levels are maintained for longer. And it relieves inflammations and protects the body against inflammatory immuno-response diseases such as arthritis.[30]

Although short-lived, its highly unsaturated nature also has the effect of fine-tuning the nerves, passing messages more efficiently. It helps to regulate calcium metabolism, depositing as much of this mineral as is needed in the nerves for its excitory function, while assisting in depositing the rest safely in the bones. PGE1 is responsible, too, for ordering the thymus gland to generate T-cells to destroy invasions by threatening alien matter. Finally, it opposes the last stage of the linoleic acid pathway which sees the creation of arachidonic acid (AA). AA creates PGE2 whose actions are pretty much the opposite of those of PGE1. It induces platelet aggregation, orders the kidney to retain salt so that blood pressure rises and causes inflammatory immune responses. At the right time, these actions are very important but often they are unnecessary and possibly damaging. An allergy to a seemingly innocuous substance, for example, is thought to have its roots in an excess of PGE2.

PGE3 is made from omega 3 linolenic acid (LNA 18: 3n-3). The LNA metabolic pathway sees it converted to stearidonic acid (SDA 18: 4n-3), eicosatetraenoic acid (ETA 20: 4n-3) and finally eicosapentaenoic acid (EPA 20: 5n-3). Found in particularly high amounts in fish oils, PGE3 works in a similar fashion to PGE1. This explains the cholesterol-regulating effect on the Eskimos' metabolism that we saw in Chapter 2.[31]

However, scientists have discovered that the first stages of these pathways are sometimes blocked – especially by free radicals and lack of enzymes – leading to a host of related deficiency symptoms. Many people now choose to circumvent this problem by taking evening primrose oil as it contains high amounts of GLA, the unsaturate that occurs after the first stage of LA metabolism. Taking essential fatty acids in the form of supplements is a subject we'll examine in Part Three.

References

1 *The Amino Revolution* Erdmann R. Jones M. (Century: London 1987) *Supernutrition* Passwater R. (Pocket Books: NY 1976)

2 *Food Allergy* (Edsell: London 1985)

3,6,10,14,20,21&23 *Fats And Oils* Erasmus U. (Alive: Vancouver 1986)

4 *Colon Health Handbook* Gray R. (Rockridge: Oakland, CA 1984)

5 *The Fat Factor* O'Mullane and Muir (Thorsons: Wellingborough 1986)

7&12 *The Chemistry of Life* Rose S. (Pelican: London 1985)

8 *The Stress Of Life* Selye H. (McGraw-Hill: NY 1975)

9 'Cholesterol in food rich in omega 3 fatty acids' Weiner M. *N. Eng. J. of Clin. Nutr*. 315 (Sept. 25 1986)

11 'Effect of dietary cholesterol and degree of fat unsaturation on plasma lipid levels' Oh S. Monaco P. *Am. J. of Clin. Nutr*. 42 (1985)

12 *The Lively Membranes* Robertson R.N. (Cam. Univ. Press: Cambridge 1983)

13. 'Nutrients that modify brain function' Wurtman R. *Scientific Am*. (April 1982)
The Chemistry of Behaviour Reinis S. Gottman J. (Plenum Press: NY 1982)

15&16 *Life Extension* Pearson D. Shaw S. (Warner: NY 1981)

17 *Ageless Ageing* Kenton L. (Century: London 1985)

18 *The Amino Revolution* Erdmann R. Jones M. (Century: London 1987) 'The basis of free radical pathology' Demopolos H.B. *Federation Proceedings* 32

19 *Brain Allergies* Philpot W. (Keats: Connecticut 1980)

22 'HDL Cholesterol is not a major risk factor for ischaemic heart disease in British men' Pocock S. *Brit. Med. J.* 292 (1986)
'Secondary prevention and lipid lowering' Detre K. et al. *Am. Health* (January 1985)
'How LDL receptors influence cholesterol and atherosclerosis' *Scientific Am*. 251 (1984)

24 *Fats and Oils* Erasmus U. (Alive: Vancouver 1986) *Life Extension* Pearson D. Shaw S. (Warner: NY 1981)

25&26 *Mental and Elemental Nutrients* Pfeiffer C. (Keats: Connecticut 1975)

27&28 *Refining of Oils and Fats* Anderson A. (Pergamon Press: NY 1962)

29 *Evening Primrose Oil* Graham J. (Thorsons: Wellingborough 1986)
The Prostaglandins Horrobin D.F. (Eden: Montreal 1976)

30 'Triene Prostaglandins' Needleman P. *Proceedings of the Nat Acad Science* (1979)

31 'Effect of different ratios of dietary n-6 and n-3 fatty acids on fatty acid composition, prostaglandin formation and platelet aggregation in rats.' Takahashi R. Horrobin D. *Thrombosis Research* 47 (1987)

Chapter 4

The Fat Revolution

So far we have explored those metabolic pathways in which fat is digested, absorbed, then reassembled inside the body. Plasma lipoproteins and chylomicrons have loomed around us like biochemical blimps; phosphatides and cholesterol have fused and then separated in an eternal metabolic courtship to maintain structural fluidity in the cells; essential fatty acids have established electrical potential, regulated plasma fat levels and provided the reactive tissue for our vital organs; and the brief sparks of life supplied by the prostaglandins have helped co-ordinate the entire, stupendously complex process.

What we should do now is see how the ever-growing awareness of the importance of essential fatty acids to the body – and the numerous sources of potential fat deficiency – are leading increasing numbers of health professionals to look to fat as a source of nutritional therapy. In this chapter we'll look at the ways in which essential fatty acids can be used to ameliorate illnesses. Illnesses, what's more, that until recently were thought to have no connection with fat at all.

Sickness out of deficiency

Nowadays, there is growing evidence and realization that ill-health comes about largely thanks to internal nutritional deficiencies. If you do not have the elements needed to support all the body's functions, then, and only then, will you succumb to illness and disease. [1] A common example cited to support this view is the way in which the health of your digestive system affects your health at large: it's all very well taking pills and syrups to clear, say, a stomach virus, the argument goes, but if the acids and enzymes in the stomach had been powerful enough in the first place, they would have destroyed the virus before it took hold.[2] Consuming medicines will succeed only in further undermining the stomach's own defences.

To ensure that the stomach is able to generate the necessary digestive chemicals means including in your diet ample amounts of all those nutrients that are used by the metabolic pathways to manufacture these enzymes and acids. Even then, you cannot be fully confident of success since there may be deficiencies in other, seemingly unrelated nutrients. This shortage will put stresses on the available substances to compensate for the shortfall, diverting the nutrients needed for your stomach defences from their proper task. Before long a pattern of deficiencies will establish itself, spiralling your health out of control. This is only one example of many. Full health, the full health of a strong immune system, and the stamina to withstand emotional and physical stress, the full health that protects you from cardio-vascular disorders and other degenerative diseases, can only be expected when your body is supplied with EVERY nutrient it needs.[3]

Rather than giving the body the nutrients it needs to help develop high levels of vitality, conventional medicine tends to use substances which work by suppressing the symptoms of illness or by directly killing pathogens. In the case of antibiotics, the medicines also kill the body's intestinal flora thereby suppressing its own defences. In those rare instances when medical authorities do recognize the importance of nutrition as a central pillar of their treatment, they focus their attentions on a dispiritingly small, select band of nutrients. The use of vitamin C, dating from the time of Captain Cook onwards, to guard against scurvy is one example. Using the B vitamins to eradicate beriberi, pellagra and rickets is another. People in certain categories today – pregnant or lactating mothers, women experiencing menstruation, older people, people recuperating from operation or illness – are given supplements of certain vitamins and minerals to guard against imbalances. But this is all so piecemeal. There is overwhelming evidence to show that these commonly used supplements barely scratch the surface, merely hint at the true extent, of the nutritional deficiencies which are crying out to be rectified.[4]

After the First World War, a Western man's life expectancy stood at approximately 70 years. Today, after almost a century of startling medical advances, the figure has risen by a paltry two years to 72. Clearly, something quite fundamental to our health has been overlooked, some imbalance has yet to be redressed. Let's track down this imbalance with a bit of detective work by examining each set of the body's major nutrients.

The indissoluble triad

Broadly speaking, our bodies are made from two structural groupings: protein structures, together with the substances that regulate them, enzymes; and lipid (fat) structures, and their regulatory substances, hormones. The two interrelate on a grand scale with each other and with vitamins and minerals to create every cell and every function in the body, coming together then splitting away in a biochemical waltz we know as the metabolic pathways. The constituents of these pathways are, in turn, divided into three categories. They are:

1. Modulators
These include antioxidant vitamins such as A and C, fat-soluble vitamins D and E, minerals such as selenium, and fibre. Modulators control the extent of chemical reactions in the body as well as protecting certain chemicals from being interfered with by others. Because of their protective properties they are often used in supplement form to provide biochemical support to a body that has been invaded by cancer.

2. Catalyst co-factors
This group includes many vitamins, particularly B complex, and minerals such as zinc, copper, magnesium and calcium. In the chemical metamorphoses of the metabolic pathways, their presence is vital for bringing one substance into contact with another, thereby enabling chemical transformations to take place.

3. Substrates
This group is composed of essential amino acids (the building blocks of protein) and essential fatty acids (the building blocks of lipids). These substances provide the underlying structures upon which the modulators and co-factors react and upon which everything in the body is built. [5]

The nutrients in these groups have overlapping and interchangeable functions. Bone, for example, thought of as a calcium structure is, in fact, a latticework of proteinaceous scaffolding with calcium phosphate attached. Enzymes may be composed primarily of protein but they need the presence of minerals and vitamins to create them. Cell walls are built of fat molecules but this fat – phosphatide – needs the presence of phosphate molecules to enable it to line up properly while calcium helps generate electrical potential for the nerve impulses in the cells created from fat and protein. [6]

As you can see, if there is a deficiency of one nutrient, the entire biochemical

51

house of cards is threatened with collapse. This is why supplements are sold and prescribed so widely. Yet most of these supplements support only the modulators and co-factors. The shelves of chemists and health food shops are crammed with the products to prove it – effervescent vitamin C, B complex, brewer's yeast, E in capsule form, chelated minerals, zinc citrate, iron. The products that support the substrate, by contrast, are tiny. A small corner of one shelf devoted to amino acids plus a packet or two of evening primrose oil. And in contrast with the others, very few people have much of an idea what these substances are for. Why is this? Simply put, because fats and proteins are present in our food in such large amounts that deficiency of these nutrients is deemed to be impossible. Is this true?

In a word: no. Admittedly, our overall intake of fat and protein is high, and has remained so for hundreds of years. However, the quality of these substrate nutrients has declined sharply. The greatest recorded decrease has occurred in the omega 3, linolenic acid, group of fatty acids. This was demonstrated graphically by a recent study which compared the nutrient intake of Eskimos on traditional diets with that of the diets of urban-dwelling Danes. The findings revealed that the availability of the omega 3 essential fatty acids in the modern diet was only 20 per cent that of the traditional intake. Furthermore, there appeared to be an almost precise correlation between the fivefold decrease in omega 3 consumption and the fivefold increase in the so-called modern diseases: diabetes, liver failure, cardio-vascular disease and cancer.[7]

These diseases, banes of modern Western society, have become prominent health threats only since the advent of the Industrial Revolution in the mid-eighteenth century. The hardship, deprivation and widespread malnutrition among the labouring classes during this period was looked upon as the main cause of diseases such as pellagra and beriberi – diseases that were supposedly eradicated in the 1930s with the widespread introduction and prescription of B vitamins – but until now very few people have associated these other, possibly even more destructive, diseases with the Industrial Revolution.

Any sense of self-congratulation at having forestalled the nutritional ravages of the revolution, therefore, is self-delusion. Whilst the malnutrition born from poverty has been largely stamped out, there have been other, less discernible, but equally pernicious effects on the standards of our food intake. And we are still paying for these today with a catastrophic heart attack rate and one death in five due to cancer.[8]

The Industrial Revolution changed not just the country's working practices but the way we treated our food – a change every bit as momentous as the more obvious aspects of this tremendous social upheaval. The advent of huge factories devoted to batch-processing food in bulk, the need to be able to store and preserve this food for long periods, and the disappearance of traditional cottage industries created a society devoted in its entirety to denaturing traditionally high-value food. Those chemicals that caused food to rot quickly were removed – never mind that they were the chemicals which gave the food its nutritional value.

Early victims of this trend towards denaturing were oils high in essential fatty acids, such as flax. Where the omega 6 and 3 polyunsaturates were not refined out, they were replaced by more stable, inert but nutritionally damaging varieties such as the lards derived from stearic acid, obtained by tallowers and renderers from the carcasses of livestock. At the same time, consumption of fresh, oily fish high in EPA, an acid in the linolenic family, saw a similar decline.[9]

Food was likewise adulterated for cosmetic considerations. Where nourishing wholemeal bread had once been a staple, it was replaced by the refined white alternative; first by the moneyed classes wishing at once to dissociate themselves from the workers and emphasize their refined palates, and then in turn by the workers wishing to emulate the moneyed classes.[10] The loss of dietary fibre (one of the body's modulators) saw the removal of one of nature's most important means of controlling metabolism of fat and cholesterol in the gut. This, coupled with an increase in refined sugar intake, meant enormous new stresses on the body when it came to coping with fat. And with the removal of the essential polyunsaturates – the molecules responsible for reducing plasma fat levels – related diseases grew enormously. (In Chapters 5 and 6 we will look at the methods of food processing in greater depth.)

Today, therefore, even when all the modulators and co-factors are in their places, as long as the diet contains largely poor quality essential fatty acids, the so-called modern diseases will continue to plague Western society. Only by ensuring that your diet is high in the entire omega 6 and 3 families can you be sure that your body is fully equipped to stave off these diseases. Now let's look at these modern diseases and see how essential fatty acids combat them.

Crimes of the heart

Cardio-vascular diseases (CVD) – heart attack; heart failure; stroke; thrombosis; high blood pressure; arteriosclerosis; atherosclerosis – are together the greatest single killer in Western civilization, causing approximately 50 per cent of all deaths.[11]

As with most diseases, its roots lie at the start of a chain reaction, each stage of which increases the potential threat posed to the possible victim. Early stages in the escalation of CVD may include a smoking habit, a diet high in refined carbohydrates and cholesterol and low in dietary essential fatty acids, and a sedentary lifestyle. The next stage, thanks to the lack of dietary modulators, will be the rapid absorption of fats and a rise in the body's plasma lipid count – increasing the number of triglycerides, low density and very low density lipoproteins and cholesterol in the blood. These in turn lead to sticky blood platelets – causing the blood literally to ooze around the body instead of flowing – scarring and hardening of the artery walls, and saturated fat tissue agglomerating in waxy clumps around the heart and on the arteries.[12]

As the space available for the blood flow shrinks, the heart has to beat harder to squeeze it into the capillaries. The combination of sluggish, slow-moving blood and vessels which dilate only with difficulty puts enormous demands on a heart whose contractions are already restricted by a straitjacket of fat. Blood pressure rises and the victim may experience the cramping pains of angina. If these warnings are ignored the blood may start to clot, causing thrombosis, stroke, coronary and even gangrene, and the heart may stop temporarily or cease functioning altogether.

Essential fatty acids can help to guard against these symptoms with three important functions. Firstly, they transport, metabolize and regulate cholesterol and other saturated fatty acids. Omega 6 gamma linolenic acid (GLA 18: 3n-6) lowers serum cholesterol up to 200 times more effectively than any other fatty acid. GLA and eicosapentaenoic acid (EPA 20: 5n-3, the fatty acid created by the elongation of the omega 3 linolenic acid, and found in fish oil) both raise the body's levels of high density lipoproteins. These are the carrier molecules that return cholesterol and other fats to the liver, prior to conversion to bile acids and subsequent deposition and excretion in the gut. This helps to inhibit the buildup of tissue fat characteristic of atherosclerosis.[13]

Secondly, as precursors of prostaglandins E1 and E3, essential fatty acids reduce the stickiness of blood platelets. They may achieve this by altering the composition of the blood cell membrane which will increase the tendency of the cells to disperse. They also reduce the levels of a blood-clotting factor, thromboxane. The result is to make the blood flow more easily, reducing the likelihood of clotting in the vessels.[14]

Thirdly, as vital structural components, they help to repair the linings of the arterial walls after the scarring of arteriosclerosis. They enhance elasticity and in turn increase the tendency of the capillaries to dilate. This ensures that blood reaches all areas of the body, carrying with it life-giving oxygen and nutrients. As high potency chemical components of the phosphatides in the membrane, they also play an important part in controlling the ion flow of the cell wall. This causes sodium to drop out of the cell, in turn reducing the cell's water content and by this means, reducing blood pressure.[15] A graphic description of the relief provided by essential fatty acids to a patient suffering from CVD can be found on pages 112 to 113.

Cancer

Unlike CVD, the effects of essential fatty acids on cancer are less clear-cut. Many tumour cells have protein receptor cells in their membranes designed specifically for docking with the fat-carrying low density lipoproteins. Therefore, whichever factors help to lower plasma LDL levels (such as essential fatty acids) could well help to retard tumour growth. However, although both omega 6 and 3 regulate fatty acid metabolism, producing HDLs in favour of LDLs, some researchers have suggested that an imbalance between these two fatty acids might actually increase the likelihood of tumour growth. What seems to be more likely, however, is that omega 3 levels are today so lacking in our diets, that regardless of omega 6 levels there is the appearance of imbalance. The fact that the last forty years have seen some stunning work into the uses of essential fatty acids on inhibiting cancer growth seems to confirm this. Let us see what this work has discovered.[16]

Protein-oil, the cancer fighter

Most of the work conducted in this area has centred on the way that fat interacts with protein. In their role as the substrates, fat and protein form the structural foundations of our bodies. They provide strength and rigidity. They also provide tensile pliancy. Since all organisms must stretch and bend as well as being firm and resistant, protein and fat could almost be looked at in the same light as the steel and concrete structure of a skyscraper – built strong enough to sustain its own massive weight, but with enough give to sway in the wind and absorb earth tremors. However, no matter how advanced the modern hi-tech office block becomes it will never be able to self-renew. Unlike living beings, whose substrate chemicals are part of an eternal self-regenerating tide, a skyscraper can't repair itself when the weather corrodes away chunks of masonry or rusts its cantilevered girders, replace broken windows, solder fuses and burst water pipes, or even redecorate its corridors and offices. It is inert and lifeless.[17] In contrast, the substrate chemicals in our bodies are partici-pating in a constant organic ebb and flow. New lipoprotein structures are continually built into old, while the oldest are broken down and carried away; lipoprotein carrier cells transport materials around the body before themselves being broken down and reconstituted elsewhere; furthermore, fat is vital for capturing the oxygen which must be burnt to provide energy to manufacture new protein structures. And all this carries on thanks to the dynamic relationship between protein and fat.

An excellent example of the intimacy of the protein-fat relationship is found by looking at the skin. Skin protein - called collagen - is an enormously complex reticulated configuration, cross-linking like a three dimensional steel-mesh fence. While it is collagen that provides the structure and rigidity of skin, fats provide pliancy and lubrication, and through their regulatory functions in the cell walls, ensure that the skin is properly fed and guarded from infection.[18] For the perfect example of fat and protein working together in this way, touch the skin of a young baby. It will be so smooth, soft and moist that it should almost feel as if you are running your finger over an expensive beauty cream. However, all too often the baby is weaned prematurely off its mother's milk - high in the essential fatty acids LA and LNA - and onto the lower quality cow's milk. Then, in consequence of this loss, the skin may become dry, flaky and inflamed, even though its source of protein is as high as before.

A fully realized combination of fat with protein, therefore, is immensely important, not just for the health of babies but for all our health. As if to confirm this, studies conducted into the effects of different nutritional regimes find that high protein diets containing very little fat - such as those followed by body builders and athletes - cause serious physical and psychological disorder. Exhaustion sets in very easily, the body falls prey to illness, and mood swings become common. Post-viral syndrome, or M.E., is very common among this group of people and the eradication of fat from the diet is thought to have a close correlation.[19] Fat and protein, therefore, as well as linking on a structural level, also participate in an important energy interchange, renewing tissue depleted by stresses such as exercise, emotional turmoil or illness. So what does this have to do with cancer?

Skimmed milk, flax and sulphur

In the 1920s, American scientist Professor Meyerhoff discovered that all biochemically intensively active tissue contains a combination of sulphur-based amino acids and dietary essential fatty acids. He discovered that administering these in supplement form to a group of athlete volunteers helped their muscles to recover much more quickly from the stress and exhaustion of intense training.[20]

This work was extended to an almost fantastic degree by the work of German scientist Dr Joanna Budwig. In the 1940s and 50s she conducted pioneering work into the causes of cancer, diabetes and liver disease – itself a precursor to cancer. She discovered that victims commonly lacked the essential fatty acids, had extremely low phosphatide levels and very little of the lipoprotein called haemoglobin. This is a protein-fat cell which the body uses to transport oxygen around the body. As cancer was seen to flourish in an environment lacking oxygen, the loss of haemoglobin might, she thought, be a major contributory factor to encouraging tumour growth.[21]

Without these important fatty acids, her patients suffered from lassitude, lack of vitality and anaemia and these factors, she thought, prevented the body from actively fighting the diseases that had invaded it. Her priority, therefore, was to raise the body's energy levels, providing it with the fuel to fight off these seemingly overwhelming stresses. Familiar with work already conducted into protein/oil combinations, she attacked the diseases in her patients with high quantities of flax oil – the richest available source of LNA – together with skimmed milk. This form of milk contains a concentrated source of LNA's most active protein companion in the substrate, the sulphur-based amino acid group. As she increased this practice, she began to achieve results almost beyond her dreams. With a rise in phospholipid levels, the vitality of her patients increased enormously. More striking was that their tumours ceased growing then began to shrink, in some cases disappearing altogether in as little as three months.

The essential fatty acids also contribute to fighting cancer in certain subsidiary ways. Most tumour cells have built-on protein receptors in their membranes to dock with LDLs and VLDL (very low density lipoproteins – the triglyceride-carrying molecules). This is more than circumstantial evidence to suggest that these lipoproteins assist cancer growth, and research has shown that the LA and LNA, by raising HDL levels and pushing down the amounts of plasma cholesterol and saturated fat, can retard and inhibit tumour growth.[22]

The loss of phosphatides – a common metabolic sign that a body is hosting a tumour – also inhibits membrane reproduction. Since cancer cells thrive in this environment – creating 'polyploidinous' cells (or many cells sharing a single membrane) – a decline in phosphatides may be a measurable forerunner of cancer. In tests, concentrations of essential fatty acids have killed incubated cancer cells and assisted normal cells in outgrowing the malignant varieties.[23]

Earlier in the chapter we talked about the ravages of modern food processing techniques on the nutritional qualities of fat. In Part Two we will look at these techniques in greater depth.

References

1 *Ageless Ageing* Kenton L. (Century: London 1985)

2 *Functional Gastrointestinal Disorders* Latimer P. (Springer: NY 1983) *Tissue Cleaning Through Bowel Management* Jenson B. (Jenson: Escondido CA 1981)

3 *Time Alive* Kenton L. & S. (Octopus: London 1988)

4&8 'Omega 3 essential fatty acids in medicine' Rudin D. *1985 Yearbook of Nutritional Medicine*

5 *Modern Nutrition in Health and Disease* Goodhart R.S. (Lea and Feibiger: Philadelphia 1973)

6 *Minerals* Erdmann R. Jones M. (Century: London 1988)

7,11,15&20 *Fats and Oils* Erasmus U. (Alive: Vancouver 1986)

9 *Food For Nought: The Decline in Nutrition* Hall R. (Random House: NY 1974)

10 *Mental and Elemental Nutrients* Pfeiffer C. (Keats: Connecticut 1975)

12 *Supernutrition for Healthy Hearts* Passwater R. (Jove: NY 1977) 'Dietary fat and blood pressure' Puska P. et al. *Preventive Medicine (Helsinki)* 14 (1985) 'Serum cholesterol response to dietary cholesterol' Hegsted D. *Am. J. Clin. Nutr*. 44 (1986)

13 'EPA and prevention of thrombosis and arteriosclerosis' Taylor T. et al. *Lancet* 1378 (1979)

14 'Prostaglandins and the cardiovascular system' Vane J.R. *Brit. Heart J.* (1983)

16 'LA deficiency in man' Holman R. *Nutritional Review* vol 40 (May 1982) *The Living State and Cancer* Szent-Gyorgi A. (Dekker: NY 1978)

17 *The Amino Revolution* Erdmann R. Jones M. (Century: London 1987)

18 *Ageless Ageing* Kenton L. (Century: London 1985)

19 *The Stress of Life* Selye H. (McGraw-Hill: NY 1975)

21 *The Basic Function of Cell respiration in its relationship to Auto-oxidisable Nutrients (essential fatty acids and sulphur-rich proteins)* Budwig J. (Hyperion Verlag: Freiburg 1953)
Light Energy in Life Processes Budwig J. (Resch Verlag: Innsbruck 1979)

22 *Diet, Nutrition and Cancer* Nat. Res. Council. (Nat. Acad. Science: Washington DC 1982)

23 'Tumour Lipids: Biochemistry and Metabolism' Wood R (Am. Oils Chem. Soc.: Champaign Ill 1973)

Part Two

Fat and Fiction

Chapter 5

Lipids and Food

Now that we understand the nature of fats and oils, this, the second part of the book, looks at the roles they play in our day-to-day lives. We shall see which food sources are highest in particular varieties of fatty acid chains, how food processing changes their natural qualities, which fats and oils to cook with, which are the best methods of cooking and which fats we should avoid at all times. We'll also contribute to some familiar debates on the subject, throwing our hats into the ring on the issue of margarine versus butter. First, let's look at the most common sources of fatty acid, essential and non-essential, in our foods.

Fats in food

Almost everything we eat contains fatty acids. After water, fat is the most abundant substance in every living thing. In animals it makes up between 15 and 22 per cent of overall body weight, compared to 12 per cent for protein, 5 per cent for carbohydrate and 3.5 per cent for minerals.[1] The cell walls of everything we eat are composed of varying levels of phosphatides entwined with protein cell receptors and structures. Phosphatides, you may remember, are trident-shaped molecules with two fatty acid prongs and a third composed of phosphate. The phosphatide/protein ratio varies enormously depending on the role of the cell. The greater the chemical sensitivity of the cell, the higher the ratio will be in phosphatide's favour. In vital organs or glands such as brain, eyeball, adrenals and testes, phosphatide levels are very high. For example, while red blood cells contain 45 per cent phosphatide to 55 per cent protein, the membranes of nerve cells contain 80 per cent to 20 per cent respectively. [2]

Not only does the phosphatide concentration rise the more sensitive the cell is, the essential fatty acids these phosphatides contain become progressively more unsaturated. This explains why non-industrialized tribes such as Eskimos instinctively choose to eat animal organs such as brain and sweetbreads in preference to the lower quality muscle meat favoured in the West. Since they contain high concentrations of essential fatty acids, these foods help to inhibit the amounts of saturated fat and cholesterol circulating in the blood. [3]

In the same way that essential fatty acids tend to concentrate in those parts of an animal's anatomy where there is greatest need for chemical reactivity, so in fresh, leafy vegetables the fatty acids predominate in the chlorophyll. It is chlorophyll that causes the single most important function in plant life – photosynthesis. This is the conversion of sunlight into energy which the plant can use for growth, regeneration and reproduction.

As we've seen, fats and oils – or lipids – are made up of the individual fatty acids contained in the foods we eat. Since most of the lipids we consume are obtained from other food sources, the quality of those lipids – whether saturated, unsaturated, trans or cis – is determined by our choice of food. As a rule, the foods from which oil can be extracted are generally the foods higher in essential fatty acids. Why is this?

Whether the lipid is a fat or oil depends on the fatty acid's melting point. This, in turn, is dictated by its degree of potential chemical reactivity. This chemical reactivity is set by whether the fatty acid chain is saturated with hydrogen atoms, monounsaturated by the absence of one pair of hydrogen atoms from the chain, creating a double bond, or polyunsaturated leading to two or more cis-configuring double bonds. The more double bonds, the greater the fatty acid's chemical potential, and the lower its melting point. To give an example, the lipid extracted from an organ of high chemical reactivity – such as cod liver – is the liquid at room temperature and therefore an oil. On the other hand, the lipid obtained from cooking a leg of beef is hard and waxy at room temperature and therefore a fat. It comes as no surprise to find that the oil in cod liver contains super-unsaturates from the omega 3, linolenic acid family, while the beef-fat is an inert, long-chain saturated fat, stearic acid. [4]

What this means in practice is that it is possible to affect your fat intake – not necessarily cutting down on fat so much as changing the nature of the fat you eat – with a few simple modifications to your diet. So now let us consider which foods contain which fatty acids.

Unsaturates and food

Unsaturates fall into three main categories – omega 9, omega 6, and omega 3. The omega number indicates where the first double bond on the fatty acid chain occurs, counting from the methyl (left) end of the molecule. The main omega 9 fatty acid is oleic acid. This is found in olives, almonds, pecan, cashew, filbert and macademia nuts. Oleic acid and its omega 9 siblings are mono-saturates which is to say that, with only one double bond, their low degree of chemical activity means that they play low-key roles in body metabolism. They contribute mainly to the structural elements of phosphatides.

In contrast the omega 6, cis polyunsaturated family is crucial for all aspects of bodily metabolism.[5] The main fatty acids in this group are:

Linoleic acid (LA). Because a healthy body can make the others in this family, it is called a parent molecule and is one of the two dietary essential fatty acids. Linoleic acid is found· in many nuts and seeds, especially flax (linseed), safflower, sunflower, soyabean, and walnut oils.

Gamma linolenic acid (GLA). This is a rare required (essential but not dietary essential) fatty acid whose best source is GLA complex which is grown from a vegetable source. Other sources include mother's milk, borage, black-currants, and evening primrose oil. Although GLA can be made from LA, we will see in Chapter 9 that this process is prone to blockage from numerous factors, and many persons suffer from acute deficiencies of this required fatty acid.

Arachidonic acid (AA). In contrast to the previous two fatty acids, a shortage of this polyunsaturate is rarely seen. It is concentrated in most of the meats people eat, and can be made from the parent molecule of fatty acid: linoleic acid (LA).

Like omega 6, omega 3 essential fatty acids are vital metabolic components. The dominant members of this family are:

Linolenic acid (LNA). Linolenic is the dietary essential fatty acid that is the parent molecule in the group, from which others can be formed by a healthy human body. This oil is found in flax (linseed), hemp, pumpkin seeds, soya bean, and walnut oil.

Stearidonic acid (SDA). Found in wild seeds. *Eicosapentaenoic acid (EPA)* and *docosahexaenoic acid (DHA)*. These are the most active of all essential fatty acids, found in fish such as salmon, trout, herring, mackerel and sardines as well as marine animals.[7]

We shall be encountering the omega 6 and 3 fatty acids many times in the subsequent chapters, discovering graphically how they enhance the body's health.

Finally, the saturated fatty acids are composed largely of three main molecules. These are:

Stearic acid (SA). This long-chained saturate is found in beef, mutton and pork. Its chemical stability and high melting point make it very dangerous to the body if the balance of essential fatty acids tips in its favour.

Palmitic acid (PA). This is a medium-chained saturate found in coconut and palm kernel oils.

Butyric acid (BA). This short-chained saturate is the largest single constituent of butter.

Having already discovered in previous chapters the relative merits of each of these fatty acids, the obvious thing to do is to eat foods high in the omega 6 and 3 families. To this end many people now cook with oils extracted from foods such a sunflower and soya beans. What could be better? We'll find out in the next chapter.

References

1 *Life Extension* Pearson D. Shaw S. (Warner: NY 1981)

2 *The Chemistry of Life* Rose S. (Pelican: London 1985)

3 *British Medical J* 291 (23rd November 1985) 'A study of the prevalence of arthritis in Alaskan Eskimos' Blumberg B. et al *Arth. Rheum.* 4 (1961)

4 *Fats and Oils* Erasmus U. (Alive: Vancouver 1986)

5 'Essential Fatty Acids in Perspective' Sinclair H. *Human Nutrition* 38 (1984) *The Lively Membranes* Robertson R. (Cambridge Univ. Press: Cambridge 1983)

6&7 *Fats and Oils* Erasmus U. (Alive: Vancouver 1986)

Mental and Elemental Nutrients Pfeiffer C. (Keats: Connecticut 1975)

Chapter 6

Refined Tastes

These days, much of the available shelf-space in British supermarkets is stocked with exotic or unusual produce. Unfamiliar fruits and vegetables appear in the greengrocery department, strange cheeses and live, organic yogurts in the dairy, squid, spices, sauces and Columbian coffee all add variety and richness to what is traditionally thought of as bland British eating habits.

Amongst this explosion of variety and choice is an ever-increasing stock of oils, margarines and butters. Grapeseed, sunflower, soya bean and olive oils stand alongside the more traditional selection of corn and other, unspecified, vegetable oils. Most of these newer products lay claim to being both cold-pressed and rich sources of essential fatty acids. They are also labelled with statistics detailing the ratio of saturate to polyunsaturate. Therefore, when the consumers see a large percentage of the oil they choose is made up of essential fatty acids, they can feel comfortable in the knowledge that they are making the correct choices of nutrition in order to enhance their health. After all, cooking with a concentrated source of one of the most important of all nutritional groups must be good.

Sadly, the truth is less wholesome. The seemingly bald statistics on the bottles camouflage a hair-raising story of adulteration and spoilage. The true picture is one of highly-mechanized industrial processes tortuously wringing the oils from their natural sources while the pressures of the market-place blithely dictate extending the oils' shelf-lives far beyond their natural spans. These twin factors mean that the products, although still technically 'high in polyunsaturates', retain only a fraction of their natural goodness.

The hard pressed facts

Once, oils were produced in limited batches by small mills found in every town. Gradually, from the onset of the Industrial Revolution, these mills have been replaced by huge, centralized factories extracting hundreds of gallons of oil a day from factory-farmed seeds. To avoid rapid spoilage the more sensitive oils such as flax have been phased out of production altogether while others have had their chemically active components – such as lecithin – removed to slow down degradation and spoilage and consequently make them more stable.[1] The effect of this on shop-bought oils is comparable to the effects of refining complex carbohydrate to produce substances such as white flour. In each case the removal of the co-factors necessary for helping the body to metabolize the products has in turn led to a rise in the incidence of fat-related diseases. There can be no more graphic illustration of the effect this loss of nutrition value has on the body than the fact that since the turn of the century, death from cardio-vascular disease has risen from 15 per cent of the population to 50 per cent, and cancer mortality from 3 per cent to 23 per cent.[2]

So let us look at the way oil is extracted, processed and sold today. Then, by understanding the effects of these procedures on our health we can actively search for alternatives.

An odyssey of refinement

In their journeys to the supermarket shelves, many oils undergo a series of refining processes that are positively operatic in their level of destructiveness. It's almost as if the oils have to surrender to various ordeals of fire and water before they can be deemed worthy of human consumption.[3]

The first stage of the refining process involves crushing the oil sources – such as sunflower and grape seeds, or the flesh and stones of olives – while cooking for two hours at an average temperature of 120°C. This has the effect of breaking down the cell walls of the source so that it is easier to extract the oils within. Bearing in mind the great sensitivity to heat of the polyunsaturated fatty acids, this will have already started causing the cis-configured double bonds to rotate, straightening the fatty acids out into the undesirable trans alternatives.[4]

The next stage involves expeller pressing the seeds or flesh of the oil sources. They are fed into huge cylinders which house screws, the edges of which fit flush with the cylinder walls. Rotating continuously, the screws drive the seeds forward onto a rigid metal crushing-head. As they are packed onto and crushed by the head, their oils are squeezed out and they run through slits in the cylinder walls to collect in massive tanks underneath. The size of the cylinder slits is adjustable. The smaller they are made, the greater the pressure becomes inside the cylinder, in turn forcing more of the remaining oil out from the pulp. Although the expeller-crushed seeds may well have been cooked before extracting the oil, the fact that they were not subjected to any specific heating process while in the cylinders means that they can be labelled 'cold-pressed'.

However, whether or not they were cooked is irrelevant. The enormous pressures and frictions inside the cylinders themselves create temperatures high enough to heat the oils. The average is between 85°C and 95°C although this will rise further as the slits are narrowed to extract the last drops of oil. The oil which is bottled immediately following the first, larger-slit, pressing – particularly olive oil – is designated as 'extra virgin'. Considering the temperatures it has weathered, it is by no means in an ideal state, but we consider it one of the best supermarket products you can buy. It retains its vitamin and mineral co-factors together with a large portion of its essential fatty acids and phosphatides. However, this oil clouds easily and it has a distinctive smell and taste. And, as it spoils rapidly is must be transported as quickly as possible to its point of sale, in turn pushing up its sale price. In contrast to these qualities, the producers want an oil that stays crystal clear, is odourless and tasteless so as not to offend the consumer, and will keep for a long time so that it can be transported at leisure and therefore sold cheaply. The lengths they will go to achieve this make the initial screw-pressings seem positively benign.

For example, any seed cake, or pulp, left over from the enormous pressures of the crushing is dissolved in a powerful solvent and agitated to remove the last of the oil. This potent mixture is then heated to around 150°C at which point the solvent begins to evaporate away leaving the oil behind. This method is sometimes used to extract oil from uncrushed seeds. No matter how thoroughly the mixture is heated to remove the solvent, some will remain to contaminate the oil.

Next, the chemicals which contribute to rapid spoilage are removed. This stage is known euphemistically as degumming. Water and phosphoric acid is mixed with the oil which is then heated to around 60°C. This drives out phosphatides such as lecithin and acetylcholine. It also ejects chlorophyll. Since each of these substances have high chemical potential and readily attract oxygen, their loss helps to prolong the life of the oil. This stage also sees the removal of mineral co-factors such as calcium, magnesium, iron and copper.

Next, caustic soda is mixed with the oil at temperatures approaching 75°C and agitated. This removes any free fatty acids present in the oil (that is, fatty acids which are not yet part of the trident triglyceride or phosphatide configurations) as well as any remaining phosphatide.

Then the oil is bleached for half an hour at around 110°C by passing it through fuller's earth or clays treated with acids. These remove the pigments. Any remaining chlorophyll is filtered out together with betacarotene. It is around this time that toxic peroxides start to form. Polyunsaturates are particularly vulnerable to attack and destruction from these substances. They set in motion a chain of free radical activity that can cross-link the fatty acids, mutating them into a variety of strange and unnatural configurations. These help to block, break down and destroy many vital chemical reactions. Peroxidation also helps to forge conjugated fatty acids – isomers such as dimers and polymers – from the essential fatty acids. Similar to trans unsaturated fatty acids, they masquerade as essential fatty acids, lining with enzymes and co-factors that are needed elsewhere and slotting into important cell structures without being able to perform actively the tasks they have taken on.

Let us take stock of what we have seen so far. The oil has been heated, adulterated with acids and alkalis and subjected to enormous pressures. The nutritious phosphatides and essential fatty acids have been either leached out or mutated into unnatural configurations, while the co-factors have disappeared altogether. And at each stage the oil has been in contact with the air, reacting with oxygen in the presence of the heat and pressure catalysts to degrade further. By now, not surprisingly, the oil stinks. To compensate it undergoes its final stage – deodorization. Here, under pressure, the oil is steam-distilled at temperatures approaching 270°C for up to an hour. If any cis-configured fatty acid hasn't yet rotated on its chain, like a chicken on a spit, into its trans counterpart, now is its big chance.

What also comes as a shock is the realization that this oil still qualifies as cold-pressed. Furthermore, to gather the information for the label, the polyunsaturate content of the oil is measured from clinical laboratory conditions using oil freshly extracted from the seed. For a clearer picture of the fatty acid content, it should ideally be tested after undergoing the industrial refining processes. As it stands, the polyunsaturate content declared on the label will often bear little relation to the healthfulness of the bottle's contents.[5]

Back on the shelf

Now the process is finally complete and the newly sanitized oil sits on the supermarket shelf waiting for the consumer to snap it up. Having read this chapter and determined not to buy such oil, he or she passes along the shelf until coming to the pure virgin olive oil. Bearing in mind that it has been subjected to a far milder form of processing, is it worth buying? Well . . . perhaps and perhaps not. Since it is so much less adulterated than its counterparts, it is more vulnerable to degradation. So let us consider what measures the producers have taken to protect it from this. If it is in a transparent container than it has been penetrated by light, creating free radicals, peroxides and cross-linkages. If in a plastic container rather than glass it might also have become contaminated with polyvinylchloride – a toxic residue of the plastic's manufacturing process. In order to prevent the chemical activity caused by light it is advisable to buy oil in an opaque container. Even here, though, there are certain pitfalls since some tin containers allow small amounts of lead to leach out from their soldered seams.

When all is said and done, the best bet is to buy traditionally pressed oil from the local health food shop. Preferably it should be stored and thus purchased in an opaque or tinned container. If the bottle is transparent, then once at home it should be stored in the refrigerator in anything that will block out the light – a small cardboard box will do. If the oil starts to cloud while in the fridge it is nothing to worry about. On the contrary, it is a sign that it still retains important nutrients. Some destructive factors are impossible to avoid, however. Every time the lid is removed for example, the oil is exposed to the potential ravages of freshly circulating air. For this reason it makes sense to buy the oil in small amounts.[6]

Now the consumer is home at last, safe behind the front door away from the predatory machinations of the food producers. Now to start cooking with oil fastidiously chosen from the many available. It is at about this time that even the most die-hard health watchers will be tempted to throw up their arms in despair and reach for a gallon bottle of industrial quality vegetable oil. Why? Because, very simply, oil which is high in polyunsaturates is not good for cooking with. While it is delicious as a dressing on salads, the presence of the chemically active essential fatty acids means that when used for frying, it will rapidly degrade. Reacting with the heat and oxygen, it produces an assortment of trans fatty acids, peroxides and free radicals. In fact, provided you use small amounts, it is better to cook with oils containing short chain saturated fatty acids such as butyric acid (butter) or palmitic acid (coconut oil). Although they perform no important tasks, and in large amounts are metabolized in the body to form the more damaging longer chain saturates, their comparative stability means that they won't react adversely with the air and heat.

If you do decide to cook with your high-polyunsaturated oil then follow a few simple pointers: put the food you wish to fry in the oil before heating. This was a traditional Chinese stir-fry method that today is largely neglected. Alternatively, before heating, you could add some water to the oil. This will help keep the temperature of the oil sufficiently low to prevent the formation of large numbers of trans fatty acids while simultaneously forming a mist of vapour above the oil surface to protect it from contact with the air.[7]

Buying food inevitably presents a dilemma to the health-conscious consumer. Whether to decide on the easy option and purchase and prepare food which may not be so good for your health but is at least convenient; or insist on the highest health standards and cook only with those foods rigorously chosen for their ability to enhance your health and vitality. The choices are not made any easier by the fact that the results of your choice, whatever it is, are never immediately apparent. You won't immediately start to suffer from illnesses of fatty degeneration if you choose unwisely, neither will you suddenly develop new levels of well-being if you choose well.

Another classic kitchen dilemma is the battle between butter and margarine for the hearts and minds of the consumer. This battle raises important health issues and it is these that we shall examine in the next chapter.

References

1&5 *Refining of Fats and Oils* Anderson A. (Pergamon Press: NY 1962)
Fats and Oils Erasmus U. (Alive: Vancouver 1986)
2 *Nutritional Yearbook of Medicine* Rudin D. (1985)
3 *The Poisons Around Us* Schroeder H. (Keats: Connecticut 1978)
4 'Trans Fatty Acids – metabolism and nutritional significance' Gurr M. *Nutritional Bulletin* 47 (1986)
6 *Brain Allergies* Philpott W. (Keats: Connecticut 1980)
7 *Fats and Oils* Erasmus U. (Alive: Vancouver 1986)
Food oils and their uses Weiss T. (Avi: Connecticut 1983)

Chapter 7

What Eight Out of Ten Consumers Should Know

Nowadays, companies wishing to increase their market share of sales in a particular product can turn to two distinct forms of product promotion. One is advertising, the other public relations. In essence, advertising consists of buying space in the various forms of media – television, colour supplements, billboards and so on – and using this space to display the client's product as enticingly as possible. Public relations is more oblique in its approach. Using a clever mix of strategies – contentious and surprising survey results, promotions that give away holidays or cars, feature articles that purport to represent an objective overview of the product or industry – public relations is primarily about making editors of influential magazines and television programmes devote space or air time to the product.

The reasoning behind public relations is that when potential buyers of the client's product see seemingly objective editorial space being used to say how good that product is, they are more likely to be swayed into buying it than by seeing an obviously subjective advertisement. Most people would be shocked by the amount of material in newspapers, magazines and on television generated by public relations activity in this way. Most PR exercises are fairly obvious and quite harmless: the sudden appearance of an actor or writer on all the chat shows is bound to herald a new film or book, for instance. Other campaigns, though, can be insidious and extremely harmful.[1]

One public relations company, for example, recently chose to promote a well-known brand of chocolate bar by stating that the bar was better for you than an apple. The company achieved this feat very cleverly, obtaining a spectacular amount of 'impartial' press coverage for the chocolate bar in the process.[2]

The method it employed was simplicity itself. A retired doctor was hired to stamp his name on a medical study, conducted under supposedly rigorous scientific standards, which claimed that apples are bad for your teeth.

This conclusion was arrived at on the basis that the pith and flesh from an apple sometimes lodges between your teeth. If left untended it will oxidize to form corrosive acids that may eventually degrade the enamel. The chocolate, on the other hand, is made of soluble material and will be washed away by the normal process of salivation. Therefore, the chocolate bar is deemed better for you. QED.

The absurdity of deeming the bar, with its unearthly content of refined sugar, denuded of fibre, vitamins and minerals, as superior to an apple, crammed as it is with all these nutrients, went largely unchallenged. What seemed to count was that the survey, blessed with the approval of a man of science, had given such an assertion this air of respectability. Of course, the story, carefully released to selected journalists, received sensational coverage. It had the front pages of several tabloids, extensive features in women's, diet and health magazines and even a television spot. Such was the *brio* with which it was conceived and executed that those in a position to refute the survey's findings were taken off guard so that their complaints sounded like the harpings of misguided health 'fanatics'.

Having read the story in a glossy magazine, what is a parent, beset by noisy kids who prefer colourfully packaged sweets to staid old fruit to think? If the magazine suggests that chocolate is good after all why not give in to the kids' demands and let them have some?

This story gives an insight into the lengths that food producers will go to market their products. It has been cited because PR of this kind is a weapon that margarine producers have been using for many years with spectacular results. Since the war, sales of margarine have risen dramatically, driven by a brilliantly conceived marketing plan that stresses the fact that they are high in the nutritionally essential polyunsaturated fatty acids. Butter manufacturers, on the other hand, have been frozen in a state of permanent defence, desultorily pointing out that their produce contains no more calories than margarine. Even the fact that butter tastes so much better has been disputed by advertising quoting the proverbial eight out of ten consumers who couldn't tell the difference.

Of course, the margarine marketers are not lying when they stress the polyunsaturate content. Most products – particularly the sunflower margarines – are high in these fatty acids. Butter, in contrast, contains almost pure saturated fatty acid. But, just as with the chocolate bar–apple issue, when you start to examine the scientific basis behind the claims, the picture is nowhere near as clear-cut. Having looked at the issue ourselves we are throwing our hats into the ring with three possibly contentious statements:

- in small amounts butter is better for you than margarine
- in amounts large or small, the trans fatty acids in most margarines are a form of metabolic poison
- butter may be not only highly nutritious but an underexploited form of alternative health therapy

Now let's explain the reasons for making these seemingly sweeping statements. A good place to start is by listing the indisputable, totally objective scientific facts.

Butter

Almost 80 per cent of the fats in butter are saturated. Of this, nearly half is made of short-chain fatty acids. Butyric acid, the four-carbon-chained fatty acid which derives its name from butter itself is the main constituent in this group with a small percentage comprising six, eight and ten carbon-chained fatty acids. Palmitic acid (PA 16:0) makes up a further 35 per cent and stearic acid (SA 18:0) nine per cent. Of the unsaturates, around 20 per cent is composed of the monounsaturated oleic acid (OA 18: 1n-9). Butter contains almost no omega 6, linoleic fatty acids – a cursory 2 or 3 per cent – and absolutely no omega 3. It contains some cholesterol (0.05 per cent) and some quantities of vitamins, minerals and amino acids.[3]

Margarine

As margarines are derived from fatty acids such as those obtained from the oils of soya beans and sunflower seeds, many contain a large proportion, perhaps 60 per cent or over, of the essential polyunsaturates, linoleic and linolenic acid. They also contain some long-chain saturates such as stearic acid. Margarine contains no cholesterol but also has no essential nutrients.[4]

Unravelling the controversy

It's astonishing how, from these few, simple, incontrovertible facts, such contradictory viewpoints have evolved. It has to be conceded that the weight of argument seemingly lies with margarine. Butter is almost wholly crammed with saturates – and we know how dangerous they can be to your health – while margarine has a high polyunsaturate content. A subsidiary argument in margarine's favour is that, since butter is made from cow's milk, it will inevitably contain traces of the hormones and antibiotics that are regularly fed to cows to stimulate greater milk yields and stave off infections respectively. When we ingest the antibiotics they will kill off some of the friendly bacteria, such as bifidus, that we carry around with us in the gut to assist with digestion. This will stimulate the growth and resistance to unhealthy varieties such as Candida albicans. Meanwhile, the hormones are thought to play a part in blocking the delta 6 desaturase stage of metabolism of LA and LNA to the prostaglandins. [5]

All in all, the margarine companies would seem to be holding all the cards. Still, let us pause for a moment and take a considered look at the way margarine is manufactured. The word 'manufactured' is used advisedly, as even the companies themselves would admit that the entire process is one of high-technology, super-efficient automation.

As we saw in the last chapter, recovering the oil from seeds is a process that has little respect for the fragility of the nutrients it contains. The enormous pressures resulting from the industrial batch-processing – crushing, bleaching, deodorizing, cooking and refining – all play their part in degrading the nutritional quality of the oil. Let us assume, even then, that this oil retains a good proportion of its essential fatty acids intact and arrives ready to be converted into margarine. The most common process the oil next has to undergo to make it solid is known as hydrogenation – and herein lies a tale. [6]

The unsaturated torture chamber

Hydrogenation is a process that takes an oil – preferably a cheap or degraded oil but any will do – and gives it a 'user-friendly', spreadable texture. Hydrogen

76

is introduced to the oil and, with the catalysing effects of intense pressure, high temperature (up to 210°C) and a metal oxide, the two are blended together to form a fat. The final consistency of the product depends on the degree of hydrogenation. Complete hydrogenation means that all the available double bonds in the fatty acid chains have become saturated with the newly introduced hydrogen atoms. Products resulting from this include lard and shortening. Their dull, heavy textures give a clue as to their chemical reactivity: they are lifeless. They have long shelf lives, and can be used for frying, baking, or roasting without any of the side effects that we saw on page 71 when polyunsaturates are cooked with. In large amounts, of course, they also help to raise the plasma cholesterol levels and should be avoided wherever possible.[7]

Most margarines are created from partial hydrogenation. The exceptions are margarines made completely by emulsifying the cis-forms of vegetable oils with medium-chained saturated fats, e.g. Vitaquell. These have none of the toxic effects of margarines made by hydrogenation. If linoleic acid (18: 2n-6), for example, were to be fully hydrogenated, it would become stearic acid (18:0). Partial hydrogenation, though, interrupts the process before it is complete, leaving a host of partly unpredictable intermediate stages. For example, the high pressures and temperatures cause the cis fatty acid's double bonds, originally all on the same side of their molecule, to rotate and face each other from opposing sides. The action of the double bonds in repelling each other then causes the molecule to unkink itself, forming a trans fatty acid. The molecule is, in effect, being tortured into disfigurement. Furthermore, their own naturally highly reactive states enhance and compound the transforming effects of the chemical action.[8]

Hydrogenation is the cornerstone of margarine manufacture. Even the margarines that claim to be high in polyunsaturates, containing, for example, unhydrogenated sunflower oil (a good source of linoleic acid) will contain 10 per cent of more of trans fatty acids to give margarine its waxy consistency.[9] This texture is due to the tendency of trans-configured fatty acids to stack very closely together and to their concomitant higher melting point. Since the melting points of trans are so much higher than those of cis, the extent of unsaturation is a highly misleading guide to its health-giving properties.

Trans fatty acids are absorbed as easily through the mucosa as their cis counterparts. However, once in the metabolic pathways, they only partially fit into the enzymes and membranes of the body and, in doing so, block the cis molecules from assuming their proper positions in structures such as phospholipids. Although most people do not recognize the cause, the consequences of this substitution are severe: the integrity of the cell membrane will be reduced, admitting substances such as allergens, undigested foods, viruses and even potential carcinogens. And the metabolic pathways of the omega 6 and omega 3 families will be blocked, preventing the creation of other essential fatty acids such as gamma linolenic acid and reducing the level of prostaglandins in the body.[10]

As cis essential fatty acids are crucial components of the body's lipid regulating mechanism, when they are substituted by the dysfunctioning trans fats, this mechanism may be seriously diminished. Trans fatty acids have been found to raise serum lipids such as cholesterol and have a bearing in the incidence of atherosclerosis, Several reports also indicate that trans fatty acids also inhibit delta-6-desaturase activity – the reactions that elongate, and add extra double bonds to, the omega 6 and 3 essential fatty acid families to forge the prostaglandins. This leads to a series of 'rogue' prostaglandins that may lead to inflammation, higher blood pressure and glandular dysfunction. In hard margarine, between 18 and 36 per cent will consist of trans, in soft margarine, between 8 and 21 per cent, while in butter, the level is between 1 and 7 per cent, much of which can easily be metabolized.

To emphasize the danger of trans fatty acids, the Dutch government – typically one of the more enlightened of European governments – recently passed legislation banning the sale of margarines containing trans fatty acid products. The only similar product which they are happy to sell is one created in Germany which emulsifies the oil rather than hydrogenates it.

The final word on the subject is left to Herbert Dutton, one of the most respected and experienced voices on fat metabolism in the world. Speaking of the dangerous effects of hydrogenation, and the problems which we now know it causes, he said: 'If the hydrogenation process were discovered today, it probably could not be adopted by the oil (food rather than fuel) industry.'[11]

What about the contrast between butter and margarine in cooking? As butter is composed largely of saturates, it makes a stable cooking medium. Furthermore, since the butyric acid carbon chain is so short, if it is consumed in small amounts, a lot of the fat will be burnt off as energy. Some cooks complain that when fried or used to roast vegetables, it burns too easily. Since its carbon chain is so short this is quite understandable. Nonetheless, with an imaginative culinary repertoire, you can do wonders with butter. Purified butter – or ghee – for example, is a staple of Indian cooking. Margarine, on the other hand, while making a convenient alternative – particularly in cakes and puddings where its soft texture blends easily with flour – is not recommended. In cooking the margarine, the remaining cis fatty acid content that has survived hydrogenation will be twisted into a toxic trans configuration.[12]

Finally, even if no other recommendation could be found, butter, unlike margarine, has been a natural dietary staple, used instinctively by human beings for thousands of years. And it's usually when we set aside our instincts and tamper with what is natural that the danger arises. Take bread, for instance. Until the near-eradication of wholemeal bread by the fashionable milling processes of the late eighteenth and early nineteenth centuries and its replacement by white bread, wholemeal flour was one of butter's natural allies. White bread, on the other hand, is denuded of the fibre, vitamins, minerals and essential fatty acids – all of which are crucial for regulating the metabolism of butter fat. Unrefined food has an 'inbred ability' to assist the body in assimilating foods such as butter. We saw in Chapter 4 that every available nutrient is needed to ensure that every other can perform its designated function, otherwise even the most benign food can become a threat, or even the most efficacious fail to improve the body's vitality.

Speaking of vitality, it's now time to look at some oils which no one disputes are among the most important and health-enhancing dietary substances on earth.

References

1 *The Waste Makers* Packard V. (Pelican: London 1977)
2 Personal experience of author
3,4,10&11 *Fats and Oils* Erasmus U. (Alive: Vancouver 1986)
5 *Chemical Children* Mansfield L. Monro J. (Century: London 1987)
6 *Refining of Oils and Fats* Anderson A. (Pergamon Press: NY 1962)
7&8 *Fettfibel* Budwig J. (Hyperion Verlag: W. German 1979)
9 *New Health Magazine* (August 1985)
12 'Intensification of essential fatty acid deficiency by dietary trans fatty acids' Hill E.E. et al. *J. Nutr.* 109 (1979)

Part Three

The Lipid Lifestyle

Chapter 8

The Unsaturated Sea

Of the essential fatty acids, the only two which we cannot manufacture in the body are the omega 6 linoleic acid and the omega 3 linolenic acid. Since these are the precursors of every other essential fatty acid, so the reasoning goes, we only have to supply these two to our bodies in ample amounts and we shall have every fatty acid we need. However, there are a great many factors which prevent the two parent molecules from satisfactorily metabolizing to the rest of the omega 6 and omega 3 families in this way. These factors include a high saturate intake, too many trans polyunsaturates in the diet, food additives, lack of the necessary dietary co-factors, free radical activity, drink, tobacco, stress, illness and ageing.[1] Therefore, it is far better to obtain each of the other essential (but not necessarily dietary essential) fatty acids from sources in your diet. Such sources include nuts, soya beans and sunflower, evening primrose and flax oils – each of which is high in one or other fatty acid from the omega 6 and omega 3 families. However, one of the most potent of all sources of essential fatty acids is not found on land at all, but in the sea.

The essential fatty acids in the oils of many fish have remarkable health-enhancing properties. They can inhibit cardio-vascular disorders, combat psoriasis and asthma, fight cancer, and inhibit the occurrence of rheumatoid arthritis.[2]

Fish, particularly in those regions nearer our coastlines, have traditionally been regarded as dietary staples. More recently, though, as our instinctive feel for which foods are good for us has failed, consumption of fresh fish has declined dramatically. Heavily processed alternatives such as fish fingers, most of whose goodness has been thoroughly destroyed before they reach the dinner table, are these days more popular. Changing tastes and perceptions must bear the brunt of the blame for this as it is probably easier to obtain fresh fish today than it has ever been. However, unlike fish fingers, or any one of the similar carotene-coloured-batter packaged products, fish can be inconvenient to prepare; it can leave unpleasant odours in the kitchen and it may be too strong for many modern palates reared on a menu of monosodium glutamate blandness.[3] After all, when we say something smells fishy, we are not being complimentary. Then again . . .

Fresh fish and foul

The most surprising thing about eating sashimi – the exquisitely prepared pieces of raw fish on the menu at Japanese sushi bars – is the delicacy of flavour. It hardly tastes the way you expect fish to taste at all. If its qualities of creamy lightness resemble anything, they resemble butter fresh from the churn. It is the same with a trout that is gutted and cooked as soon as it has been landed by an angler. The flavour has the most fulsome of gourmets reaching for their thesaurus. However, leave the sashimi, or that freshly caught trout, to stand for a while and the flavour changes dramatically as the oil starts to degrade. Very quickly the meat begins to smell, the taste becomes richer and ranker. Although this rapid degradation is one reason why fish is not as popular as it used to be, it also gives us a clue as to why fish is so good for us.

Another clue is supplied by tasting cod liver oil. Supposedly an important nutritional supplement, particularly during the war when food was rationed, it is said to help eyesight, guard against rickets and other muscle and bone disorders and improve circulation. Yet how can these assertions be measured against something that tastes so foul? Its sour, rubbery flavour clings to the tongue and sides of the mouth, and if the recipient is unlucky enough to burp, he or she must relive the experience all over again.

The reason cod liver oil tastes the way it does is simply because it is actually rancid. Although, when fresh, it is a highly nutritious food, its packaging undermines its health value. The light-rays admitted by its clear glass bottle, the oxygen in the air which comes into contact with the contents every time the screw top is removed, and the fact that it is often kept on the shelf of a warm kitchen, all contribute to its rapid degradation. But other oils are stored in similar conditions without degrading anywhere near as quickly. Why should cod liver oil spoil so much faster?

As we have seen, oil degrades as the result of chemical activity. The more pronounced this degradation, the greater the activity. We have also seen that certain fats degrade only very slowly – these tend to be the chemically inert saturates. The greater the degree of polyunsaturation, on the other hand, the greater its instability and its tendency to react to the heat, light or oxygen. For this reason, as we saw in Part Two, a fat such as butter is better to cook with than sunflower oil. By the same token, the fact that the fish oil degrades so quickly indicates an enormously high level of chemical reactivity (try cooking with cod liver oil, and see how bad it is).[4]

This is why fish oils are so very important. The speed of degradation is due purely to two highly unsaturated fatty acids derived from the omega 3, linolenic acid group. They are eicosapentaenoic acid (EPA 20: 5n-3) and docosahexaenoic acid (DHA 22: 6n-3). As they are present in the most important chemically active tissue in the body, as well as protecting against a host of degenerative illness, they are among the most nutritious of all fatty acids. And as EPA has five double bonds and DHA six, this also makes them potentially the most chemically active of all the essential fatty acids.[5]

The best sources of these two fatty acids in nature are wild (not farmed) trout, salmon, mackerel, fresh sardines, fresh tuna, eel and cod. In these fish, EPA and DHA together constitute between 15 and 30 per cent of overall fat content where the fat itself makes up between 10 and 15 per cent of the fish's weight. As these particular species of fish are found naturally in cold, deep-water habitats, and are cold-blooded, it is crucial for their survival that the oils in their blood have low melting points and resist the tendency to agglomerate. If their blood easily becomes sticky, or clots, then they will die. With so many double bonds, however, the melting points of plasma EPA and DHA are, respectively, $-44°C$ and $-55°C$.[6] This means only at temperatures below these will the oils turn to fats.

The great number of negatively charged double bonds on these two fatty acid chains also gives them a strong tendency to repel each other and disperse. All essential fatty acids have a certain tendency to spread out, but EPA and DHA are especially good at it. So good in fact that in repelling each other, they also pull apart other, less active lipids such as saturates and cholesterol with them.[7] We can think of them roaming the blood like solitary but hyperactive police officials, breaking up groups of indolent, slovenly saturates on the suspicion of conspiracy and having each of them disperse in a different direction. EPA is also the precursor of the series 3 prostaglandin PGE3 which itself activates an anti-clotting reaction. In addition, the dilatory effect which PGE3 has on the blood vessels enhances circulation.[8]

These two fatty acids, therefore, are remarkable at making the blood more mobile and guarding against stickiness and clotting. Fish oil is also an effective hypolipidaemic agent – that is, it lowers the levels of blood triglycerides. A study conducted in 1987 at the University of Kansas administered MaxEPA (a fish oil supplement high in EPA) to a group of volunteers all of whom were from high-triglyceride risk groups. The study's results show that, although the EPA did not affect the ratio of HDL to LDL, it was significantly effective in lowering plasma levels of the triglyceride-carrying very-low-density-lipoprotein (VLDL).[9]

Another investigation, carried out in the same year in San Francisco showed that a high intake of fish oil lowered plasma lipids significantly even when the diet was high in cholesterol. This suggested 'that the fish oil was able to block the response to the added cholesterol in patients usually sensitive to dietary cholesterol'.[10]

Finally, the results of a double-blind trial of healthy volunteers at the University of Cardiff provides the most compelling evidence for the efficacy of fish oil. Sixty volunteers received supplements of either MaxEPA or olive oil for a period of six weeks, without them, or the officials conducting the study knowing which. During this time the plasma triglycerides of those volunteers taking MaxEPA decreased by 54 per cent. There was a slight increase in the overall total of serum fats but this was partly attributable to a rise in HDL, the 'good' lipoproteins that carry cholesterol and other fats away from the tissue to be dumped in the gut. The oil was also observed to prolong the blood clotting time, increasing its mobility and therefore reducing blood pressure.[11]

This last test goes some way towards explaining why Eskimos, whose diets are largely meat and blubber, enjoy such a low prevalence of cardio-vascular disease. The high levels of EPA in the fish meat they consume is at least partly responsible for their health. However, an extensive and exhaustive study conducted by the Efamol Research Institute in Nova Scotia, Canada, suggests that rather than having one cause for the low rate of heart and circulatory disorders, there may be several.

The study found that Eskimos have a genetic variation from normal essential fatty acid metabolism in that they are unable to create arachidonic acid (AA 20: 4n-6). This fatty acid, which is in the omega 6 group, is created by the desaturation (removal of two hydrogen atoms) of dihomogamma linolenic acid. AA is responsible for the creation of series 2 prostaglandin PGE2. In the right time and place, this substance is very important – it is used in allergy and immune responses. However, the same response sometimes leads to inflammation and degeneration of soft tissue. Unlike people from 'Western' cultures, Eskimos somehow manage naturally to block the creation of AA.

The study concluded that if we wished to emulate the high levels of vitality in Eskimos, we would have to raise our levels of gamma linolenic acid (GLA 18: 3n-6) into the bargain. Although in the same pathway as AA, GLA is the precursor of series 1 prostaglandin PGE1, and this inhibits the activity of PGE2. Since natural conversion from the parent LA to GLA is very slow, the best way of raising GLA levels is through a supplement of GLA complex. This particular product is a British breakthrough with high levels of GLA and as an additional benefit is the only known vegetable source of squalene, an oil that helps stimulate the immune system. GLA complex is the best natural source we know of this particular essential (required) fatty acid. [12] (We will be looking at GLA and evening primrose oil and the processes and obstacles involved in its creation in the following chapter.)

Recommending two different essential fatty acids – possibly both in supplement form – to improve the body's health potential is one example of the way that their different properties can be made to complement each other. As we learn more about the value of essential fatty acids, it is likely that supplementation will increasingly take this form. As we shall see in Chapter 11, some patients are already benefiting from the mix.

Most research conducted into the importance of fish oil has centred on its effect on blood pressure, stickiness and mobility. By lowering triglyceride levels, raising the HDL count, increasing blood mobility and helping capillaries to dilate, it is an essential part of any programme to relieve the symptoms of cardio-vascular disease and bad circulation. Many people take it in supplement form simply because they find that their hands and feet retain their feeling in the winter, instead of going numb. This, too, is due to improved circulation. Fish oil does have other valuable attributes. Let us examine them.

Transducers of life

Even more extraordinary than the mechanisms by which they improve cardio-vascular health are the roles that EPA and DHA perform in the body's vital tissue. Both these fatty acids are concentrated in the body's most sensitive areas – in particular the sex glands, the brain cells, the retina (or inner lining of the eye), the inner ear, the adrenal glands and the synapses of the nerve (which are the junctions between one nerve cell and the next). In each of these areas, a high degree of chemical reactivity is essential. The mechanisms by which EPA and DHA function are even now only vaguely understood.

However, researchers believe that the connection lies in the ability of the fatty acid chains' double bonds to capture oxygen. Since oxygen molecules provide the medium for creating the energy required for chemical reactions, this is crucial. [13]

In capturing oxygen like this, EPA and DHA become, in effect, biochemical transducers, transforming energy from one form to another, then controlling and directing it. The retina, for instance, receives energy in the form of light waves which must be converted to electrical energy before being passed as impulses along the optic nerve to the brain. The same is true of the inner ear, which converts sound waves to electrical impulses for the auditory nerve. EPA and DHA, therefore, are an indispensable link in the sensory chain between the outside and inside worlds.

While energy is used to transport messages to the brain, the brain itself consumes a tremendous amount of energy and this demand is met, in part, by the metabolic activity of the essential fatty acids. The brain, a 'local area network' of staggering complexity, communicates constantly with itself, co-ordinating, comparing and relaying messages between its millions of cells. The expenditure of energy here is massive. Although it makes up only 2 per cent of body weight, fully 20 per cent of all the metabolic activity in the body occurs here.

Sexual reproduction also depends greatly on these essential fatty acids. They are present in each hormone – such as the follicle-stimulating hormone, progesterone and luteinizing hormone – the sperm, semen and ovaries, and the passages of the sex organs. [14]

The connection with oxygen and energy transfer also helps to explain why essential fatty acids have been used by Dr Joanna Budwig (see Chapter 4 pages 57 to 58) with such success to treat cancer. The fact that several oils are used in combination – the EPA and DHA from the trout she recommends, coupled with LNA from the flax oil that she also administers – is another example of the way in which essential fatty acids can be used in tandem. (Flax oil will be discussed in depth in Chapter 10.)

Without adequate levels of these fatty acids, therefore, each of these metabolically vital functions will suffer. The body becomes prone to behavioural difficulties, impotence, infertility, stress, and sight and hearing impairments, not to mention the circulatory problems that were dealt with earlier.

Obtaining fish

Bearing in mind how easy it is to obtain fresh fish, and fish oils, it is well within our powers to ensure that we have healthy levels of EPA and DHA. However, much of the wet fish on sale today has been spawned and reared in special hatcheries and farms. This is particularly so with trout. Inevitably, because the food they are fed contains little or none of linolenic or omega 3 fatty acids, the quality of the fatty acids of fish that grow in these environments will not be as high as wild or 'free range' fish. In fact this could be easily remedied by including linseed or flax seed mash in the food. Set against that is the fact that these fish will almost certainly reach your fishmonger faster than species landed from trawlers, many of which are kept in the trawlers' huge freezer containers for weeks after being caught. Either way, the wealth of essential fatty acids will still be greater than that found in red meat or game.

When cooking your fish it is best to bake it. This preserves the essential fatty acids it contains much more effectively than grilling or frying. If you want to eat the fish raw, Japanese-style, make sure the fish is very, very fresh. Some people freeze raw fish before eating it to kill any parasites or beasties that might be in the fish. Ideally it should have been killed on the day you bought it. We've seen how easily fish oil degrades and eating raw fish without knowing how fresh it is is inviting an unpleasant stomach upset.

Having looked at the merits of fish, let us turn our attention to an oil that we met briefly earlier in the chapter: gamma linolenic acid (GLA).

References

1 *Ageless Ageing* Kenton L. (Century: London 1985)

2 'Fish oil consumption and decreased risk of CVD' Herold P. *Am. J. Clin. Nutr.* 43 (1986) *New Eng J. Med* 316 (1987)

'Fish oils in rheumatoid arthritis' *Lancet* (September 26 1987)

'Fish oils as medicines' Jones R. *Lancet* (September 12 987)

3,6&11 *Fats and Oils* Erasmus U. (Alive: Vancouver 1986)

4 *British Medical Journal* 291 (23 November 1985)

5 *Life Extension* Pearson D. Shaw S. (Warner: NY 1981)

7&13 *Chemistry of Life* Rose S. (Pelican: London 1985)

8 'The effects of dietary intake of essential fatty acids on prostaglandin and leukotrine synthesis' Higgins G. *Proceedings of the Nutr. Soc.* 44 (1985)

9 Evening primrose oil, marine fish oil and CV risk factors Shreeve C.

10 'Marine oils and thrombogenesis' Dyerberg J. *Prog. Lipid Res* vol 21 (1982)

12 'Low prevalence of CHD, psoriasis, asthma and rheumatoid arthritis in Eskimos' Horrobin D. (Efamol Research Inst; Kentville, Nova Scotia, Canada) *Medical Hypotheses* 22 (1987)

14 *The Amino Revolution* Erdmann R. Jones M. (Century: London 1987)

Chapter 9

The Mother's Milk Oil

Mike, a self-employed electrical contractor, works from his home in the town of Stow-on-the-Wold, England, in the Cotswold Hills. His job often involves driving considerable distances to building sites, farm-building conversions and renovations where he will install the wiring or conduct a safety survey. One evening, after a particularly tiring day, he was driving home in his van along an unfamiliar, winding minor road. 'It was dusk; you know those few minutes around lighting up time when it's dark enough to need headlights but not dark enough for them to illuminate the road effectively.'

In his mirror he watched a car draw up behind him. From the way it kept weaving out into the middle of the road, the driver was obviously impatient to pass – a feat rendered impossible by the winding road and high hedges hiding the sight of oncoming vehicles. Perhaps Mike was watching the car behind when he should have had an eye on the road ahead, or perhaps the fact that the car was tailgating him made him accelerate. For, rounding a sharp bend much too quickly, he found himself about to crash into the rear end of a slow-moving truck. He braked violently. 'I felt the back end of the van begin to slew sideways and the truck's red tail lights shoot towards the windscreen. Still, I slowed down just in time and thought I'd got away with it.' A split second later a jarring concussion snapped through his van as the car behind, itself unable to stop in time, ran into him.

The damage wasn't great: the driver who hit him stumped up the insurance for repairs, and the minor cricked neck that Mike had suffered was expected to fade. It didn't. Instead the pain grew progressively worse, spreading along his right shoulder and down to his elbow. 'It was a horribly sharp pain that came and went,' he said. 'At times it was so bad, I couldn't move without sweating buckets from the agony of it. The doctor ordered an X-ray and put me in a collar and sling but he couldn't find anything wrong. He thought that the whiplash might have trapped a nerve. He prescribed some painkillers and a course of cortisone injections.'

When these had no effect, Mike was left at a loss. 'I couldn't drive to work so I lost money that way. When I did manage to get in, the shoulder was so bloody painful, I was afraid to move my arm even to pick up a pair of pliers.' This continued for more than two months. Then, while sitting once more in his doctor's waiting-room for a repeat prescription of painkillers, he saw an article in a much-leafed women's magazine about gamma linolenic acid (GLA). 'Most of what these things print is pretty unbelievable but then I saw that this oil was being used to treat muscle and bone complaints. I went into the doctor and asked him about it. He was a bit sceptical but didn't think it would do any harm so he gave me a prescription for a month's supply of the oil.'

After taking the capsules for less than a fortnight, the pain and immobility had completely vanished. Mike continues to take GLA capsules to this day, not because of any lingering disability, but simply because they make him feel healthy. 'I'm clearer headed, need less sleep and my circulation is better than it's been for years. Working in these half-built houses, I swear my joints used to freeze up, get so stiff. Now they're like a piano-player's fingers.'

Mother's milk in the evening

The GLA complex mentioned earlier is the only source of GLA that is remotely similar to the fatty acid profile in mother's milk. The increasing use of GLA, whether obtained from the premium source of GLA complex, or its companion product of EFAPLEX in which it is combined with omega 3 oils, or the more widely known evening primrose oil, is a classic case of the health food industry stepping in with a natural food where conventional medicine fears to tread.

Although GLA has been actually consumed for centuries in the traditional diets of Eastern people, it has come to prominence only in the past 10–15 years. Perhaps the main reason is the myth that American Indians have exploited its therapeutic powers for centuries. What is difficult to believe is that this small yellow flower seed could yield such a nutritious oil. In fact the seeds contain such small amounts of oil that huge quantities of seeds would have to be consumed to obtain anything near the required level available in capsule form.

Comparison of Human Breast Milk, GLA Complex and Evening Primrose Oil.

Oil	Human Breast Milk	GLA Complex	Evening Primrose Oil
GLA and others	22.4%	19.5%	9.0%
Palmitic	22.6%	23.5%	6.5%
Stearic	9.2%	6.5%	2.5%
Oleic	35.0%	39.5%	8.0%
Linoleic	10.8%	11.0%	74.0%

Additionally, the tested levels of GLA measured in commercially available capsules of evening primrose oil fluctuate dramatically.

Apparently, what the American Indians did use was the roots and the leaves of evening primrose plants. Indeed, GLA is such a nutritious oil that it can be used to assist the body in coping with a surprisingly wide assortment of ailments ranging from damaged nerves, as in Mike's case, to period pains and even heart disease and diabetes. In contrast with the vegetable source of GLA complex which is grown with uniform and high yields of GLA, primrose seeds mature at different rates. If harvested by hand, the source can become quite expensive. Once the oil is extracted, it is difficult to store and can turn rancid. The essential fatty acids react with light, oxygen and warmth causing the oil to degrade rather rapidly. The variables mean that the standard of quality of evening primrose oil cannot be guaranteed, even though it is carefully packaged in those gelatine capsules so readily available in health food shops and chemists. The British alternative to evening primrose oil, GLA complex, is the only source that competes with mother's milk for its content of the essential (required) gamma linolenic acid. Since few of us have ready access to mother's milk, we favour the GLA complex as the best source.

However, if human milk is the main natural source of GLA, what stops each one of us from suffering a deficiency of this essential fatty acid once we are weaned off the milk and onto a dairy alternative? The answer is that although GLA is an essential fatty acid, like the fish oils, EPA and DHA, it is not a dietary essential. This means that it can be manufactured in the body from another source. The source in this case is the categorically dietary essential, omega 6 linoleic acid (LA 18: 2n-6).

As we have seen, linoleic acid is the precursor, or parent molecule, of a number of other essential fatty acids. Through a combined process of desaturation (in which hydrogen atoms are removed to create additional double bonds) and elongation (where extra carbon atoms slot into the carbon chain), linoleic acid produces in turn gamma linolenic acid, dihomogamma linolenic acid (DGLA 20: 3n-6), and arachidonic acid (AA 20: 4n-6). (This polysyllabic metabolic pathway is known colourfully as the *arachidonic cascade*.)[3]

Of these separate, increasingly complex essential fatty acids, GLA produces series 1 prostaglandin (PGE1) while arachidonic acid produces series two prostaglandin (PGE2). At least, they do in an ideal world.

However, in this real, far from perfect, universe, the first stage of this metabolic pathway, creating GLA from LA, is often prone to blockage. The enzyme required to bring about this first-stage conversion is called delta-6-desaturase. It latches onto two adjacent hydrogen atoms on the linoleic acid chain and removes them, leaving the fatty acid free to form an additional double bond and increase its chemical potency.[4]

We saw briefly in Chapter 8 how the metabolic pathway from the parent essential fatty acid to EPA can be blocked easily, and the same holds true for the creation of GLA from LA. Like a country innocent roaming at night in an unfriendly city, the desaturase enzyme is vulnerable to a horde of violent attackers which lie in wait for it – in this case, fat-related substances. Excessive levels of plasma cholesterol, long-chain saturates and monounsaturates work to block the enzyme. And trans-polyunsaturates will, in effect, deceive the enzyme into reacting with them instead of their healthy cis counterparts. This misdirects, and wastes, much of the enzyme's limited supplies. Alcohol blocks the enzyme's production. So do deficiencies of important enzyme co-factors such as zinc, B3 and B6 which result from inadequate nourishment and consuming too much refined and processed food. High carbohydrate and sugar intake, diabetic conditions, liver disorders and ageing all prevent this enzyme from creating GLA.[5]

Therefore, even if your intake of linoleic acid is itself sufficient, there are many factors to prevent the body from progressing to the next stage. Which is where GLA in supplement form comes in. After your mother's breast milk, the highest concentration of gamma linolenic acid is found in GLA complex, followed by blackcurrant, borage, and evening primrose oil.[6]

Mistaken identities

Many people understandably confuse GLA (18: 3n-6) with the body's other great dietary essential fatty acid, omega 3 linolenic acid (LNA 18: 3n-3). As we saw in Chapter 8, LA is the precursor of the fish oil EPA (see Chapter 8) and prostaglandin series 3, PGE3. GLA and LNA have the same number of carbon atoms and double bonds. Both are cis-configured. Where they differ is that while GLA's three double bonds are situated on its sixth, ninth and twelfth carbon atoms, LNA's are found on its third, sixth and ninth. From Chapter 1 onwards we've seen how seemingly insignificant changes in the way molecules are constructed have huge ramifications for the way the body uses them. Because of this difference in the position of one double bond (twelfth against third), GLA and LNA are used for many different purposes and functions. We shall discuss LNA further in the following chapter. In the meantime, what of the effects on the body's metabolism of a readily available supply of GLA?

GLA therapy

Unlike many nutritional therapies which have originated in the 'alternative' health world, GLA is starting to become widely accepted in conventional medical circles. Efamol, a commercial product that has been around much longer than our favoured GLA complex, has been administered in large quantities to patients by the more open-minded doctors and researchers for some time. Rigorous double-blind tests – in which neither patients nor officials know whether the substance being administered is evening primrose oil or another unsaturated oil such as olive oil – have helped compile a long list of potential therapeutic uses.[7] This has in turn complemented and supported the nutritionally based exponents of the oil. Let's see some of the ways in which it is now used.

GLA can lower blood pressure. It may do this in several ways. As a component of numerous phosphatides, GLA helps to increase the pliancy of artery walls and reduce the tendency of blood cells to agglomerate.[8] They also help to form high density lipoproteins (HDL) which reduce plasma cholesterol and saturate levels.[9] As the precursor of PGE1, GLA reduces blood stickiness and allows capillaries to dilate more efficiently. Consequently, GLA oil sources are today administered widely to help combat the symptoms of CVD.[10]

As well as reducing the levels of plasma lipids and ensuring that fat is more effectively regulated, it has also been found to reduce the amount of insulin required by diabetics to regulate their blood sugar levels. This in turn reduces the stresses on a diabetic's liver and pancreas and although by no means a cure, goes a long way towards making his or her life more tolerable.[11]

GLA's ability to enhance cell pliancy, regulate fat levels and reduce stress on the liver also explain why it is used to treat alcoholics. As we saw on page 40, alcohol has the effect of making the cell wall initially more fluid. This leads to a loss of co-ordination between the protein nerve-message receptor – experienced as drunkenness – as well as damaging the membrane. To compensate, the body injects the wall with a reinforcing dose of cholesterol. This hardens the wall and enables the receptors to communicate properly. However, if alcohol is consumed regularly in large amounts, the cell walls get so saturated with cholesterol that they become permanently hardened. This in turn leads to behavioural and physical problems – such as the dreaded delirium tremens or shakes – as the receptors are once more prevented from communicating effectively.

In time, the victim is forced to drink alcohol simply to get his cell walls to a normal level of fluidity and escape the shakes. The paradox of having to drink in order to stay sober helps to explain the pernicious nature of alcoholism. It is an underlying cause of the disease and the success rate of shock treatments which force the alcoholic to give up without helping to reduce the level of cholesterol is very low. However, with gamma linolenic acid to reduce the amounts of cholesterol entering the cell wall and to assist with removing the cholesterol to the gut, recovery is often much smoother, less traumatic and ultimately more successful.[12]

Schizophrenics have been found to suffer from low levels of PGE1, and GLA has been given to assist in raising them. Some improvement has been noted, particularly in those patients who have had the disease for less than five years.[13]

This fatty acid has a 90 per cent success rate in helping reduce the symptoms of pre-menstrual disorders. These include breast pain, pre-menstrual tension, sensations of bloatedness and seemingly causeless depression and irritation.[14] One victim who, month after month, had endured black, almost suicidal depression, was delighted to find the symptoms fade simply by taking two capsules of gamma linolenic acid a day in the week before her period.

One particularly impressive feat is the way in which GLA can combat severe rheumatic and arthritic disorders. PGE1 is very successful at reducing the inflammation around joints that causes rheumatism. Many factors lead to this. One is the way in which it suppresses abnormal autoimmune responses – or allergic reactions. Wheat allergy, for example, is thought to lie at the root of many diseases including rheumatism. PGE1 helps to mitigate this reaction by instructing the thymus gland to produce a series of white blood cells called T-suppressors and they literally suppress the response.

Bone joints, more so than any other part of the body, demand a high degree of cushioning and lubrication to guard against wear and tear. A loss of these factors leads to arthritis. One of the main guarantors against this wear and tear are the synovial capsules – gelatine sacs that fit between the bone heads. GLA has an acknowledged role in maintaining their health and pliancy.[15]

The oil also improves hair condition, reduces the tendency of some nails to split and relieves eczema and psoriasis.

A note of caution when taking GLA in any of its supplement forms, though. As the body needs co-factors to metabolize the GLA on its journey along the metabolic pathway that creates PGE1, it is sensible to take these co-factors as additional supplements with the oil capsule rather than expecting your body to have sufficient amounts in store. The main co-factors are zinc and vitamins C, B3 and B6.[16]

As more and more uses are found for GLA, it seems set to storm the barricades of the health establishment at the vanguard of a movement towards more natural forms of treatment. It had better be quick about it, though, because another oil is even now starting to re-emerge into the limelight after years of neglect to challenge its eminence. It is this oil that we will meet in Chapter 10.

References

1 *Fats and Oils* Erasmus U. (Alive: Vancouver 1986)
Evening Primrose Oil Graham J. (Thorsons: Wellingborough 1985)
New Health Magazine (August 1985)
2 *Life Extension* Pearson D. Shaw S. (Warner: NY 1981)
3 'Regulatory function of delta 6 desaturase key enzyme of polyunsaturate synthesis' Brenner R. *Function and Biosynthesis of Lipids* (Plenum Press: NY 1977)
4 *Ageless Ageing* Kenton L. (Century: London 1985)
5 'Trans Fatty Acids – metabolism and nutritional significance' Gurr M. *Nutrition Bulletin* 47 (1986)

6 *J. Lipid Research* (Bethesda MD)

7 Efamol Institute: Nova Scotia, Canada

8 'Comparative effects of LA and GLA intake on plasma lipids and platelet phosphatides in elderly people' Veriel R. *Nutritional Research* (1987)

9 'Why do polyunsaturated fatty acids lower serum cholesterol?' Beynen A. *Am. J. Clin. Nutr.* 42 (1985)

10 *Clinical Uses of Essential Fatty Acids* (1st Efamol Symposium) (Eden: Montreal 1982)

11,15&16 *Fats and Oils* Erasmus U. (Alive: Vancouver 1986)

12 *Fats and Oils* Erasmus U. (Alive: Vancouver 1986)
The Lively Membranes Robertson R. (Cambridge Univ. Press: Cambridge 1983)

13 *Psychodietetics* Cheraskin E. (Bantam: NY 1974)
Mental and Elemental Nutrients Pfeiffer C. (Keats: Connecticut 1975)

14 'Effects of nutritional supplementation on pre-menstrual syndrome – double blind crossover trial' (PMS Advisory Service: Hove 1987)

Chapter 10

Flax – The Nutritional Oil-Rounder

Imagine the scene at a village cricket match on a green in Kent. It is late in the afternoon one summer Sunday. The sun dips below the row of ancient oaks lining the green and the shadows of the cricketers, whose white flannels are streaked with grass stains, lengthen towards the picket fence on the far side. A small crowd of onlookers has gathered beneath the trees, sitting in striped canvas deckchairs or leaning languidly against the gnarled trunks, somnolently transfixed by the last over of the match. The home team, which is batting and down to its final two batsmen, needs three runs to clinch the game. Defeat is almost assured, since the over is to be delivered by the visitors' demon bowler (figures: six for nine). Holding their collective breath in anticipation, the fielders crouch around the batsman's wicket and the bowler sprints in like a bloodcrazed tartar. One final ranging stride jams his leading foot into the popping crease, the momentum windmilling his arm over the bails. With a grunt of expelled breath he releases the ball. It hits the wicket slightly short of a length, and rears up at the batsman like a striking cobra. The man ducks, hoisting his bat instinctively to shield his temples. The crack of leather on willow pierces the twilight and the ball glances away to the boundary, to score a four. There is a murmuring of applause and the players leave the field to the sound of nightingale song from the darkening sky.

What does this have in common with fats and oils? Look at the match-winning batsman as he walks towards the wooden pavilion, his cheeks flushed red from his exertions and exposure to the late afternoon sun. Held under his arm like a sergeant major's baton is his bat, a yard of sturdy willow, cracked at its base and with the binding on the handle coming adrift. The day before, our hero retrieved this ancient bat from a cobwebbed tomb in his attic,

99

nervously eyeing the cracked face. The bat appeared dry and brittle. When he knocked a ball, the wood made a hollow sound, and the impact stung his fingers. Out came his can of linseed oil. As he rubbed the oil into the grain with a cloth, the wood seemed almost to drink it in, seemingly swelling with health before his eyes and acquiring a fresh glow of golden nut brown. Playing a few practice shots, the contact of bat and ball sounded clean and resonant. A new tensile strength in the wood easily absorbed the concussion of cork and leather against the bat, saving his fingers from any further stinging. The bat was transformed by the oil.

Aside from its use on cricket bats and as a thinning and drying medium for oil paint, linseed oil isn't given much thought. As a food it is given almost none. Yet now, an increasing number of respected nutritionists are suggesting that linseed oil may be one of the most potent sources of essential fatty acids it is possible to find. What it does to the cricket bat, they say, instilling new life and vitality into the tired wood, it will do for your state of well-being. [1]

Bought in its pure, fresh form, or alternatively obtained from newly crushed linseeds grown in fortified soil, this oil is one of the most nutritious, health-enhancing and biochemically active foods you can buy. It is used to combat cardio-vascular disease, cancer, liver and gut disorders, skin complaints, and impairment of the immune system. [2]

Naming names

Linseeds and linseed oil are obtained from the seeds of the flax plant. To distinguish between the oil used nutritionally and the lower quality derivatives used for industrial purposes such as paint dryers and wood lubricants, nutritionists prefer to call it flax oil. Flax seed and oil production once flourished throughout Europe thanks to thousands of local presses. [3] Its qualities are praised as far back as the fifth century BC in the writings of Hippocrates, the father of medicine, who discovered that it contained potent therapeutic qualities for relieving diarrhoea, gut ailments and dry skin. Mahatma Gandhi stated, 'Whenever flax seed becomes a regular food item among the people there will be better health.'

The Latin name for flax is *Linum usitatissimum* meaning 'most useful' and it is easy to see why it was so named. As well as yielding such a nutritious oil, flax is a major force in the textile industry. Once the flax has been stripped and crushed, the resulting fibrous residue is woven to make linen.

Inevitably, flax oil production declined as large industrial concerns superseded the smaller, cottage-based industries. As with most oil production, quality was sacrificed to the demands of bulk yield and what was once a staple in many people's diets was generally forgotten.[4] Now, though, thanks to the growing awareness of how closely nutrition relates to health, flax oil is making an impressive comeback. Today, the flax plant is grown in many countries around the world, from Argentina to Poland. The only areas where conditions are utterly unfavourable for it to grow are the poles and tropics. In soil whose mineral content hasn't been denuded by the high concentrations of phosphates and nitrates in synthetic fertilizer products, flax may grow to over three feet in height, flowering with sky-blue petals. The plant flourishes particularly well in slightly harsher climes, and many yield almost 50mg of oil from every 100mg of seed. When fresh, this oil has a light, delicate texture and a pleasant, nutty flavour.

Flax facts

Flax oil owes its metabolic effectiveness to the fact that it is the world's richest natural food source of the omega 3 essential fatty acid, linolenic acid (LNA 18: 3n-3). Between 50 and 60 per cent of the overall oil content of flax is composed of LNA compared to only about 2 per cent in fish. The remainder consists of 15–25 per cent linoleic acid (LA 18: 2n-6), around 20 per cent oleic acid (DA 18: 1n-9) with the rest made up of 16 and 18 carbon chain saturated fatty acids.[5] The presence of such large quantities of essential fatty acids means that it directly affects almost every aspect of the body's metabolism.[6] Unlike some biochemically active fatty acids, however, it contains substances such as carotene (or pro vitamin A) and vitamin E which help to slow down the oxidation process and thereby regulate the speed with which the flax is digested and metabolized. Such controlled metabolism means that even when taken in large amounts as a food supplement – as an increasing number of nutritionists now recommend – it will not overbalance the metabolic pathways in which it operates.

Flax is also very high in those chemicals which control the metabolism and distribution of lipids in the body. In particular, it carries large amounts of phosphatides and lecithin which, as we have seen, are essential in building and maintaining cell structure and mobility.

Phosphatides, for example, are essentially the multi-functional brickwork of the cell wall. They are arranged, like bricks, in an orderly repeating fashion but, unlike bricks, are slightly fluid to enable the cell to expand and contract. Without this fluidity, muscles would be unable to flex, skin unable to stretch. Remember how the addition of linseed oil improved the tensile strength of the cricket bat. Since phosphatides have a negatively charged phosphate chain in the third prong of their molecular tridents (resembling in all other respects a triglyceride where the third prong, like the other two, is composed of an electrically neutral fatty acid), the phosphate ensures that neighbouring phosphatides repel each other. This is a crucial feature of the molecule since it prevents the fatty acids from agglomerating in large, sticky clumps. Instead, it makes them disperse, spreading out in a thin layer across the cell wall while forming in an orderly, repeating, brick-like arrangement. This layer forms the semi-permeable skin of the cell. And, since the second, central, prong of the phosphatide is made of an essential, cis-kinked fatty acid, the resulting structural fluidity is what allows the membranes to move, rotating the protein structures embedded in the membrane wall so that they can perform their duties precisely – these include secreting enzymes, distributing food, generating immune responses to viruses and passing nerve messages in the form of electrical impulses to exactly the right area. [7]

Another of the duties of the phosphatides is to attract oxygen. Since bacteria flourish in low-oxygen, or anaerobic, environments, a shortage of phosphatides will contribute to an increase in the presence of bacteria. Similarly, since phosphatides determine the selectivity of the membrane in allowing in, or refusing entry to, foreign substances, a deficiency may lead to an increase in the penetration of carcinogens.

Phosphatide deficiency will cause the cell to be inadequately nourished, lead to behavioural disorders, cardio-vascular and skin diseases and reduced immunity – to name but a few. Phosphatides are so important that any deficiency will cause the organism to die, which is why flax, since it is a good source of these molecules, makes such an important nutrient.

Lecithin, another major component of flax, is hardly less important to the body. As the parent molecule of choline it is responsible for the lipotrophic factor, the way the body fully metabolizes its fats and oils. Since it is an 'edible detergent', it keeps blood cholesterol soluble, thereby guarding against the buildup of fatty plaques on the blood vessel walls. This could in turn lead to arteriosclerosis, high blood pressure, fibrillation and angina. It is also vital for assisting the liver in its blood detoxification function. [8] When you realize that an underperforming liver is a forerunner of cancer, choline's importance to your body becomes clear.

Lecithin will also strengthen the body's power to resist disease by acting as a metabolic precursor to prostaglandin PGE3 in the thymus gland. This short-lived regulatory molecule stimulates the thymus into producing T-cells - the body's cellular light infantry division - which will seek out and destroy virus infections.

Flax also contains a chemical that works with PGE3 to control dilation of the body's blood vessels and to assist with the withdrawal and deposition of calcium in the bones and its metabolism in the cells.[9]

Since flax oil contains so many essential nutrients, and is preternaturally high in LNA, it affects more areas of the body's metabolism than any other oil - superseding even the more widely known evening primrose oil in its metabolic potency. It is so high in those chemicals - phosphatides, lecithin, and the precursors to PGE3 - which, if included regularly in the diet, would help guard against and increase resistance to a variety of diseases - that it cried out to be used simply as a supplement to the diet for preventive purposes.[10] One area of nutritional therapy that is giving particular cause for optimism, however, is the way that flax is being used to combat a disease that no one is certain how to prevent - cancer.

Flax and cancer

A number of studies carried out over the past 20 years into the effects of essential fatty acids on cancer have focused on the way that a series of chemical compounds called *lignans* are thought to reduce the risk of contracting the disease. Lignans are produced from metabolic pathways whose parent molecules include highly unsaturated fatty acids.[11]. Quite simply, the higher the level of lignans measured in the patient's urine, the less likely statistically he or she is to fall prey to breast or colon cancer. Lignans tend to be found in greatest concentration in the urine of vegetarians.[12] In laboratory tests using rats, these compounds were shown to exert anti-tumour and anti-oxidant effects, inhibiting both the growth of cancerous breast cells and the production of carcinogens in the gut. One of the reasons suggested for this is that lignans - especially one called enterolactone - reduce the body's natural oestrogen secretion. Since cancer cells contain structures that act specifically as oestrogen receptors, many scientists believe that oestrogen actually stimulates the growth and reproduction of cancer. Lowering the level of oestrogen in a person at risk of, or suffering from, cancer, may cause a reduction in the rate of division of cancer cells.[14]

Since lignans found naturally in plants seem to have a greater effect on cancer than those made in the body from the natural processes of gut fermentation, scientists have analysed a variety of vegetable sources to discover which plant contains the highest concentration of lignans. Flax seed, it was discovered, produces 100 times more urinary lignans than its nearest competitor, wheat bran, in a test that also included soya beans, barley, corn and buckwheat. [15]

Another theory for the effectiveness of flax in fighting cancer is that it is a natural regulator of triglycerides and saturates. It will break down long-chain saturated fatty acids in favour of short-chain equivalents such as butyrate and acetate. Both these have been shown to significantly suppress the growth and division of cancer cells. [16]

Flax is also a crucial element in cancer treatment at Dr Budwig's clinic. In Chapter 4, we saw how Dr Budwig's methods centre on the relationship between the body's fatty acids and the sulphur-based amino acids, and how they produce the energy that literally powers our life. [17] Each one of the body's reactions needs this energy – it is required for something as simple as blinking an eyelid, to the multi-disciplined co-ordination of driving a car, the physical demands of a marathon or the debilitation of fighting cancer. These are all stresses and everything your body does is, to a greater or lesser extent, a response to stress. Stress is a three-stage process: an alarm where the stressor is identified; a response in which the effort is made to carry out the appropriate action to meet that stress; and exhaustion where there is no longer the energy to continue responding. The more fuel the body has, therefore, the longer the stress response can be sustained.

This fuel is provided by a 'battery' consisting of the highly unsaturated cis fatty acids containing the negative charges which, when brought into contact with the positively charged sulphydryl components of the proteins, creates the power for the stress response. They are, in effect, the two elements – anode and cathode – of the stress battery, powering our every living act. The classic example of this theory is the way that the woman's egg, which is high in essential fatty acids, is fertilized by the man's sperm which is composed largely of sulphur-based amino acids.

Dr Budwig discovered that the greater the stress put on the body – and in this context stress may mean heat, cold, tiredness, the pressure and demands of work, money troubles, emotional difficulties, injuries, burns, illness, operations and even inadequate nutrition – the faster the battery will be used up. Working on from this, she realized that as these varieties of stress take their toll – and we are under constant siege from them – we become increasingly vulnerable to all manner of degenerative diseases and, in particular, cancer.[18]

Accordingly, Dr Budwig treats her patients by establishing them on a strictly rigid diet that excludes all fats except for 100g of flax a day, which gives perhaps 50g of LNA, and trout together with a combination of raw fruit and vegetables and wholegrain products. The sulphur-based amino acids she provides in the form of skimmed milk. Using this method, Dr Budwig has achieved extra-ordinary results – supercharging her patient's life-batteries. In many cases the flax has actually helped to dissolve the existing tumour.

Dr Budwig does not use nutritional supplements herself in her practices but they are employed by others with remarkable success. A graphic example of how effective flax is when used with such supplements is demonstrated by the achievements of the Medabolics clinic in Tunbridge Wells, England. Lilly, a women of 60, visited the clinic last year with her husband to investigate the potential benefits to cancer sufferers of a regime of nutritional supplementa-tion. As a cancer victim herself, her curiosity had been sparked by the fact that the clinic had used combinations of amino acids, minerals and vitamins to assist cancer sufferers. The reason for her visit lay in the fact that four years earlier a malignant lump had been removed from her breast. This had been followed up with a course of radiotherapy. At the time, her consultant had decided that chemotherapy, with all its debilitating and disspiriting side-effects, was unnecessary.

Lilly takes up the story: 'About a year after the treatment, the lump grew again. It became terrifically inflamed and painful and the doctor presented me the choice of undergoing chemotherapy or risking full-blown cancer.' It says much for her presence of mind that she decided calmly to investigate the alternatives before embarking on a course of chemotherapy. Reading an article on the benefits of high levels of minerals, vitamins and free form amino acids and the way they strengthen the body's metabolic pathways led her to the clinic for nutritional therapy.

'When I was told of Dr Budwig's pioneering work and its philosophy of com-bining essential fatty acids and proteins, I was delighted with the simplicity of the philosophy and the way it seemed to make such good sense.' She embarked on a highly concentrated course of flax and sulphur-based aminos backed up with other supplements to strengthen her immune system. Within two weeks an improvement in the state of her lump was discernible and her overall health and physical appearance also improved tremendously. The angry swelling in her breast became quiescent after a month, shrinking to a tiny fraction of its former size. Subsequent check-ups carried out over an eight-month period revealed that chemotherapy was no longer necessary. Seemingly, when the body has adequate nutritional support it can heal itself without recourse to outside interference.

Flax elsewhere

Of course, such is its efficiency and versatility that flax is currently being used for a variety of other therapeutic purposes. Since the fatty acids it contains play a major role in maintaining the structure of cell membranes, it has been used with considerable success to treat skin afflictions that have resulted from a loss of cell membrane integrity. The membrane works like an immensely complex valve mechanism, determining both the amount and nature of the substances that enter. In this way it maintains the required amount of water inside the cells – water which is needed for many reasons including keeping the concentrations of the minerals potassium and sodium at the required levels for maintaining electrical potential. Enough water is needed to keep the cell turgid. Too much will cause the cell wall to burst, too little will make it wither and die. Any deficiency in the function of the cell wall caused by a loss of essential fatty acid (EFA), therefore, will be catastrophic.[19]

Such deficiencies are common causes of skin disorders such as eczema and psoriasis. Consequently, flax is used widely to counteract them. Studies conducted recently in Italy show that flax oil helps skin to become softer and more sensitive, while chapped lips and areas of dry skin may disappear altogether.[20] Indeed, certain suntan oil manufacturers even include flax in their products. This makes a lot of sense as the sun has the same effect on the oil in your skin as it will on the oils sitting in bottles on the supermarket shelves – namely, oxidation and rancidity. By guarding against these effects with flax oil your skin has a much better chance of surviving its annual ritualistic bake.

Flax also relieves constipation and generally assists bowel movements. Thanks to flax, movements tend to be larger and more frequent but do not cause diarrhoea. This is partly due to the lubricant action of the oil but can also be attributed to the fibre content of the linseeds which is how many people prefer to take flax[21] (means of preparation are discussed later in the chapter).

Flax oil will also regulate the body's levels of triglycerides and thereby assist in relieving the problems of liver disease. Flax has a tendency to produce short-chain fatty acids such as butyrate and acetate in the colon, both of which put fewer demands on the liver and lead to the production of fewer toxic by-products.

In addition to the high linolenic acid, flax oil is also high in the essential amino acids (that is, those elements of protein which the body is unable to manufacture and which act as precursors to the other elements), vitamins and minerals. Since adequate levels of these nutrients would, if included regularly in the diet, act as a powerful safeguard against disease, flax can be regarded as an all-in-one super-nutrient [22]. Flax has recently been given to lactating mothers and it produced softer skin, higher omega 3 content in their milk and more contented babies.

A good deal of research into the effect of flax on animals has also been carried out. American nutritionist Paul A. Stitt[23] reported a test where flax seed grown from fortified soil was administered to a group of horses. After three weeks their coats developed a beautiful sheen with their dandruff all but disappearing. Similar tests were carried out on poultry and pigs, showing a dramatic improvement in the presence in the meat of the omega 3 fatty acids. Adding flax to the diets of these animals makes a great deal more sense than feeding them with the nutritionally low-grade, bacteria-ridden mixture of ground feathers and excrement that is the norm today.

Obtaining flax

There are many brands of flax oil on the market but unfortunately few are manufactured to the required standard. It is easy to tell if the oil is good or not since, when fresh, it has a light consistency and a delicate, nutty taste. As with all oils it should be bought in an opaque glass or plastic container to protect it from the oxidizing effects of light, stored in a cool place and consumed within three weeks.

There are several ways to consume fresh flax oil. It can be added just before serving to warm dishes such as porridge, soup or sauces. Alternatively, it can be used as a dressing on your salad with, or instead of, extra virgin olive oil. It can also be taken with fruit juice. Put one tablespoon of fresh orange or lemon juice in a glass, float one tablespoon of oil on top by pouring it in carefully over a spoon, then, having added more fruit juice on top, drink it down in one draught. Since the double bonds in the fatty acids react powerfully when heated, flax should never be cooked.[24]

If you cannot obtain a good supply of linseed oil, use the organically grown seeds as an alternative. They are sold by most good health food or wholefood shops. One tablespoon of oil is equal to around three tablespoons of seeds. Ensure that the seeds you buy are whole and not split or lightly crushed. Both of these methods of presentation are common when sold in branded and sealed packets. Ideally you should crush the seeds yourself no more than twelve hours in advance of consumption. To crush them, either put them through a food grinder, add to liquid and liquidize in a blender or put in a freezer bag and lightly crush with a rolling pin. Linseeds may also be soaked overnight to form a gelatinous mass which can then be added to muesli or porridge. Make sure you chew the softened seeds to enable the digestive juices to get to the oil.

While any organically grown linseed (flax seed) should be suitable, there is an expensive (and perhaps the best) source of flax seed that comes from near the North Pole. It is called Mega Omega, in which some zinc and vitamin B6 have been added to the ground-up seeds. Normally, this would cause the oils to oxidize quickly, but these seeds are special and have enough lignans to protect the oil. So far, the powder preserves the oil for up to two years. We feel it is the best one available, but very expensive.

We believe that the best flax oil presently available in bulk comes from a Canadian company which has developed special pressing equipment, which they have patented, to make sure the extraction of the oil is carried out with low pressures and low temperatures. It is truly a cold pressed oil, done in the presence of Argon gas to make sure no oxidation occurs. Finally, it is bottled in small, hard and opaque plastic bottles which are refrigerated. If frozen, the flax oil (linseed oil) is edible for up to one year of storage. It is increasingly available through consumer demand in health food stores and from private practitioners who know of its superior qualities. You will know by now that its name, Omega Nutrition, comes from the omega oils it contains.

Again, we turn to Britain, for what we believe to be the ideal and handiest combination capsule. EFAPLEX combines emulsified flax seed oil (linseed) with some GLA complex in a single capsule. This combines the best of both families of omega oils in an easy-to-take form: no messy loose oils. Additionally, this capsule contains a vegetable source of squalene. While EFAPLEX is available only through practitioners, there is a roughly similar product, called Nutri-oil, available through health shops.

References

1 'Fats That Heal, Fats That Kill' Erasmus U. *Healing Newsletter* 22–23 (Gerson Inst: CA)

2,6,22&23 'Efficacy of feeding flax to humans and other animals' Stitt P. (Presentation to the Flax Institute Conference Fargo: N Dakota)

3,5,21&24 *Fats and Oils* Erasmus U. (Alive: Vancouver 1986)

4 *Bailey's Industrial Oils and Fat Products* Swern D. (Wiley and Sons: NY 1979)

7 *Phosphatydilcholine* Peters H. (Springer Verlag: NY 1976)

8 *Ageless Ageing* Kenton L. (Century: London 1985)

9 'The role of essential fatty acids and prostaglandins' Crawford M. *Post Med. J.* 56 (1980)

10 'Prostaglandins and the cardiovascular system' Vane J. *Brit Heart J* (1983)

11 Adlercruetz H. et al. *Lancet* 1295 (1982)

12 Adlercruetz H. *Med. Biol.* 59 (1981)

13 Horowitz C. *Nutr. Cancer* 16 (1984)

14 Lederoq G. *Bioch. Biphys. Acta* 560 (1979)

15 Axelson M. *Nature* 298 (1982)

16 *Diet: A Professional Guide* Anderson J. (1979)

17 *The Amino Revolution* Erdmann R. Jones M. (Century: London 1987)
The Stress of Life Selye H. (McGraw-Hill: NY 1975)

18 *Der Tod des Tumors* Budwig J. (Budwig: Freudenstadt 1977)
Das Fettsyndrom Budwig J. (Hyperion Verlag: Freidburg 1959)

19 *The Chemistry of Life* Rose S. (Pelican: London 1985)
Lively Membranes Robertson R. (Cambridge Univ. Press: Cambridge 1983)

20 'Essential Fatty Acids in Perspective' Sinclair H. *Human Nutrition* 38 (1984)

Chapter 11

Case Histories

We have already seen a number of cases, interspersed throughout the other chapters, of the way in which fats, and especially essential fatty acids, have rectified illnesses. In this chapter we'll look at some more.

One of the difficulties in ascribing the recovery of a patient to the use specifically of essential fatty acids is that usually when treating victims of a particular ailment, the cause is assumed to lie in a deficiency of a cross-section of nutrients rather than one particular substance. Treatment, therefore, includes several important vitamins, minerals and amino acids as well as the fat. In some cases this makes it hard to claim that the patient's recovery is thanks solely to the qualities of the fatty acid.

A good example is the way in which essential fatty acids are used to treat psoriasis – the painful itching and inflammation of the skin. Both flax and evening primrose oils have been used with enormous success to relieve these distressing symptoms. However, the important co-factors, zinc and vitamin B6, are usually administered with them as they help to metabolize the fatty acids' respective metabolic pathways. As both zinc and B6 possess skin-healing properties of their own, it's hard to say which nutrient effects the improvement. Of course, the whole point about taking co-factors is that it is the separate nutrients, interreacting as a whole, that have the effect rather than as individuals.

All the same, essential fatty acids do have very specific, highly individualized functions and the way these can be exploited to good effect is the point of this chapter. Simply remember that a deficiency of one nutrient is usually accompanied by shortages of others and that it is always wise, if taking an essential fatty acid supplement, to include its co-factors with it.

Glasnost and fish oil

Jonathan, 45, is the managing director of a small software firm in Slough, deep in the heart of England's 'silicon valley'. In his job, in one of the world's most competitive fields, he expects frequent periods of concentrated pressure. Over the past eighteen months, largely thanks to the economic changes in Russia brought about by perestroika, he has been negotiating a deal with a government technology committee in Moscow to supply his highly specialized software. This has involved numerous flights to Helsinki and Moscow, and gruelling bargaining sessions long into the night with his Soviet counterparts – accompanied by copious amounts of vodka and blinis. Running parallel with these negotiations have been others with bureaucrats in Whitehall to secure the permits necessary for exporting the technology to the Eastern Bloc. Capping this monumental juggling act is the need to keep the entire process secret from his competitors, most of whom are much bigger than his own company. Were they to get a whiff of the deal he is setting up, they would instantly mobilize a spoiling operation – using contacts in government to obstruct the licence approval while themselves making overtures to the Russian authorities. 'This period has been the worst of my life,' says Jonathan, 'I can't remember when it hasn't been ticking over in my mind. I suffer from insomnia because of it and it is affecting my health dreadfully.'

Indeed, for in the middle of the wheeling and dealing, Jonathan began to suffer from debilitatingly high blood pressure. It was measured at 156/114. The upper safety limit is considered to be 140/90. 'Spots would appear before my eyes like miniature exploding fireworks. I'd feel faint, my heart would be beating incredibly heavily, almost ponderously, as if it were twice its normal weight.' Jonathan was prescribed drugs to control the problem but, while bringing down his blood pressure, they had 'an unacceptable effect' on his sex life. 'I relish the pressures of my job. Equally I enjoy life with my wife. We have an active and fulfilling sex life and it struck me as absurd that if I wanted to experience one, then I was barred from experiencing the other. That surely wasn't right.'

Of course, there was no reason why he should be denied either, assuming his diet contained each of the nutrients needed to support his metabolism against the stresses he was experiencing. However, as he revealed when he came for nutritional counselling, his diet was far from ideal. Jonathan was a good three stone overweight and it was easy to see why. He ate foods high in saturated fats – pork, beef, and fried food in particular – together with large amounts of refined carbohydrate and sugar, and plenty of alcohol. He ate little complex carbohydrate such as wholemeal bread, no fibre of any description and no foods that could be counted as rich sources of fibre and cis-polyunsaturates. When his blood was analysed it was found to be abnormally high in low density lipoproteins. He was heading for a serious cardio-vascular disorder.

The most important step in reducing his blood pressure and helping him to avoid the potential heart disease was to establish a nutritional regime high in essential fatty acids, together with the relevant co-factors. Together they would work to regulate the levels of plasma lipids. At first, Jonathan was shocked at the idea of cutting out foods of which he was so fond. 'I might have occasionally eaten a lobster at a restaurant,' he said, 'but the idea of eating seafood instead of meat twice or three times a week was repellent at first.'

Although herring contains one undesirable fatty acid, herring, trout, cod and mackerel featured particularly high on his new menu in order to boost his intake of EPA (see pages 83–90). Since it was impractical to expect him to eat fish every day, he was also given supplements of marine fish oil capsules. These raise plasma HDL count, reduce the tendency of blood to agglomerate, and clean out the arteries. Capsules were preferred to bottles because, as we saw on page 71, the transparent glass allows in light and the screw top lets in air, both of which degrade the oil very quickly. In the first fortnight of treatment, he was also given a source of gamma linolenic acid.

On his return visit a month later, his blood pressure had sunk to well within normal range – 136/88. This had been achieved without recourse to his prescription drug and in the middle of the most stressful and gruelling time of his life. Four months later, incidentally, the deal was signed and a new one is now in the offing.

Flax and the gut

In contrast to Jonathan, who had to undergo a crash course in the importance of sound nutritional practices, Miriam, a 56-year-old, is herself a health practitioner. She runs a small mail order business selling vitamins and minerals, and her vitality was generally very high. Her one problem was that she had enormous difficulty with the health of her colon. At times she was immobilized by sharp, stabbing pains in her gut, at others it was a wearying, dull ache. She was tested for Candida albicans – the virulently damaging strains of yeast that have become a major health risk – but the results were negative. She suffered alternately from constipation and diarrhoea and when she noticed blood in her stools, she feared she might have cancer of the colon. Happily, this, too, proved negative.

When she came for nutritional counselling, the source of Miriam's problem soon became apparent. Over the previous 20 years, as a means of keeping her weight down, she had progressively eliminated all sources of fat and oil from her diet. She used fresh tomatoes on her bread rather than butter or margarine. Although she ate fish she always discarded the skin as it contained the highest concentrations of oil. Nuts, red meats and most dairy products except for low-fat yogurts were excluded to avoid the feared calories. She ate lots of fruit and vegetables but avoided wherever possible fatty or starchy produce such as avocado. She also took lots of mineral and vitamin supplements to compensate for any shortfall she might suffer as a result of excluding so much from her diet.

Obviously, while knowledgeable about the co-factor chemicals, it had not struck her that their full health-enhancing potential would never be realized without taking the substrates – particularly the essential fatty acids – into account. At first she was horrified to be told that her problem was shortage of fat preventing the gut wall from being lubricated satisfactorily. The pain and bleeding she had experienced was due to the hard stools scraping their way along the gut lining and causing inflamed and scarred pockets of tissue called diverticulitis. Periodically, her gut would attempt repairs, first purging itself by secreting extra mucus and this she experienced as diarrhoea.

As a therapy, she was put on a course of two separate fatty acids. One was flax. At first it was administered as oil in large amounts – as much as six teaspoonsful a day. Later she took it in the form of fresh flax seeds which she crushed immediately before use and sprinkled on her muesli. The flax helped to lubricate and soften the stools so that they passed more easily and eradicated the punishment on the gut wall.

Secondly, she was told to eat some butter with her bread rather than the customary tomato. The butyric acid it contains is recognized for the regenerative effects it has on the gut wall. Although the butter on its own – especially when eaten in reasonably small amounts – would be unlikely to cause weight gain, she was advised to take a little light exercise to make sure that any excess was burnt off.

When she revisited five weeks later, she had no more complaints about her gut pains and problems. Furthermore, having informed herself about the characteristics and value of certain saturated and polyunsaturated fatty acids, she had started to stock them in her own business for her customers.

The fuel-injected immune system

Sarah, 23, had been plagued continually by a series of minor illnesses since her mid teens. These were primarily cold symptoms such as sore throats, headaches, blocked nasal passages and sinuses, and mild muscle pains. Occasionally they would blow up into a major bout of influenza, knocking her out for days on end. 'If there was talk of an impending flu epidemic, then there was no way I was not going to be the first to be laid low by it,' she recalls. 'It's amazing, but it cut me off from so many normal experiences. I couldn't often taste my food, I couldn't take exercise, I couldn't socialize much with my mates because I'd always feel rotten the next morning. I wouldn't say my life was ruined, just that it was pretty dreary.'

When she came for nutritional counselling, an analysis of her blood revealed that her neutrophils – or white blood cells – were round and inactive. These cells are the mobile infantry of the body's immune system and without them, resistance to illness is greatly reduced. Healthy white blood cells are generally quite elongated and, seen under a microscope, appear to oscillate with vigour. The sluggish nature of her white blood cells meant that relatively minor viruses could invade her system which normally would be checked before taking hold.

The lack of white blood cell activity has been associated with a shortage of the chemically active phosphatide, phosphatidyl choline (see pages 43 and 102). This substance gives the cell walls the fluidity and mobility they need in order to function effectively. PGE1 and PGE3 are also required for producing healthy white blood cells. To inject her cells with the vitality to resist illness, therefore, Sarah was given supplements of lecithin, flax oil and evening primrose oil, together with the co-factor support of minerals, vitamins and amino acids. As a result, a dramatic improvement in the activity of her white blood cells was observed after only one week. Since starting this regime, she has not experienced a single sore throat, headache or case of blocked sinuses.

As essential fatty acids become widely accepted as integral components of good nutrition – rather than substances to be shunned mistakenly by individuals concerned with good health – cases such as these will become increasingly common.

Conclusion

It seems a little strange to think that this book could soon be on sale in my local supermarket, just yards from the spot where I encountered the milkmaid peddling her cracker fragments covered in low-fat spread. It is strange because they encourage attitudes towards fat which are diametrically opposed. On one side, we have the milkmaid-cum-salesperson, primed with the simple yet powerful sloganeering of her company's marketing department to exploit the customers' deep-rooted distrust of fat and its effects – drawing attention to the way fat is perceived as the cause of so many obesity-related diseases. On the other, we have this book trying to encourage a different view, showing how fat can be exploited as an immensely positive force for your health and vitality.

That fat exists at all means that it is crucial to our well-being: life is simply too harmonious a phenomenon, and too economical, to allow a substance into its complex cycles that can do nothing but harm us. On the contrary, fat fits into the metabolic pathways like a keystone in an arch. Remove that keystone and the entire edifice crumbles.

Fats play active roles at every stage of the life process. They are lubricants, cushions and insulators, guarding against the stresses, concussions and physical extremes that we encounter daily; they are transducers, converting forms of energy such as sound and light into electrical nerve impulses; they provide structural rigidity to cell membranes; and they act as taxis, ferrying harmful substances safely away from sensitive tissue. For these reasons, fat is every bit as important as amino acids, protein, minerals and vitamins.

Of course, fats can also harden arteries, raise blood pressure, contribute to cancer, diabetes and the other illnesses we've examined. But anything imbued with such metabolic power can, if misused, be a threat as well as an aid. Few people, after, all, avoid driving although cars are potentially lethal weapons –

they simply learn to drive carefully. In the same way, each one of us has a responsibility to ourselves to use fat in such a way that it enhances our health, seeing it as an essential component of our diets rather than shunning it thanks to some outdated received notions.

So next time you visit your supermarket and you happen to be approached by a milkmaid carrying a trayful of crackers, praising the virtues of the hydrolysed alternative, ignore her. Or better still lift this book from the rack, pass it to her, then carry on choosing the foods you need.

Appendix A:

Sources of Fats and Oils

Sources of saturated fats

Short chained fatty acid*
   Butryric Acid (4 Carbons) (From Butter)
Medium chained fatty acids**
   Coconut oil
   Cocoa butter
   Palm oil
   Palm kernel oil
   Cheese
   Ice cream
Long chained fatty acids
(Solid at body temperature)
   Pork
   Ham
   Lamb
   Beef
   Chicken skin
   Products such as lard, tallow, and suet
*When intake of short-chain or medium-chain fatty acids exceeds the body's need for energy, they are converted into the long-chain fatty acids and stored in the body. Once they have been converted to the long-chain fatty acids, the body can only use them for energy. They must be burned, providing calories.
**Commercially prepared baked goods, pie fillings, non-dairy cream substitutes and many fast food preparations use these medium-chain saturated fatty acids.

Table 1: Amount of saturated fat per 100g of food

Food name	Saturated fat per 100g
Nuts – coconut – raw – shredded	29.8g
Cream – whipping – heavy	23.0g
Cheese – cream	22.3g
Cheese – cheddar	21.1g
Cheese – parmesan – grated	19.1g
Bacon – broiled/fried/grilled	17.5g
Vegetable oil – peanut	16.9g
Milk – whole – dry	16.7g
Lamb – chop – lean/fat – broiled/grilled	16.6g
Nuts – Brazil – dried – shelled	16.1g
Vegetable oil – olive	14.2g
Vegetable oil – corn	12.7g
Nuts – macadamia – dried	11.0g
Vegetable oil – safflower	9.4g
Nuts – cashews – dry roasted	9.1g
Seeds – pumpkin/squash – dried	8.7g
Hamburger – beef – 21% fat	8.5g
Cheese – ricotta – whole milk	8.3g
Seeds – sesame – dried – whole	6.9g
Nuts – peanuts – spanish – dried	6.8g
Nuts – pistachio – dried	6.1g
Nuts – walnuts	5.6g
Nuts – pecans – dried –halves	5.4g
Pork – chop – lean – broiled/grilled	5.3g
Seeds – sunflower – dried	5.2g
Nuts – almonds – shelled – chopped	4.9g
Veal – cutlet – med fat – broiled/grilled	4.7g
Nut – filbert/hazel – dried – chopped	4.6g
Goose – no skin – roasted	4.6g
Duck – no skin – roasted	4.2g
Egg – duck – whole – fresh – raw	3.7g
Egg – whole – raw – large	3.3g
Roast beef – heel – lean /fat	3.3g
Ham – roasted	3.1g
Lamb – leg – lean – roasted	3.0g
Beef – liver – fried	2.9g

Sources of unsaturated fats

Although your body can make saturated fats from unsaturated fats, it cannot reverse this process.

There are several oils with a single double bond: monounsaturated oils. These come mostly from vegetable sources – legumes (pulses) and seeds. The most important monounsaturated oil is oleic acid.

Table 2: Amount of monounsaturated fat per 100g of food (all monounsaturated fats)

Food name	Monounsaturated fat per 100g
Vegetable oil – olive	73.6g
Nuts – macadamia – dried	58.1g
Nuts – filbert/hazel – dried – chopped	49.1g
Vegetable oil – peanut	46.3g
Nuts – pecans – dried – halves	42.1g
Nuts – almonds – shelled – chopped	33.9g
Nuts – pistachio – dried	32.7g
Nuts – cashews – dry roasted	27.3g
Nuts – peanuts – spanish – dried	24.4g
Vegetable oil – corn	24.2g
Bacon – pork – broiled/fried/grilled	23.8g
Nuts – Brazil – dried – shelled	23.0g
Seeds – sesame – dried – whole	18.8g
Seeds – pumpkin/squash – dried	14.3g
Nuts – walnuts	14.2g
Vegetable oil – safflower	12.1g
Avocado – raw	11.2g
Cream – whipping – heavy	10.7g
Hamburger – beef – 21% fat	10.4g
Cheese – cream	10.0g
Seeds – sunflower – dried	9.4g
Cheese – cheddar	9.4g
Cheese – parmesan – grated	8.7g
Milk – whole – dry	7.9g
Lamb – chop – lean/fat – broiled/grilled	7.6g
Pork – chop – lean – broiled/grilled	6.9g
Egg – duck – whole – fresh – raw	6.5g

Food name	Monounsaturated fat per 100g
Veal – cutlet – med fat – broiled/grilled	4.7g
Egg – whole – raw – large	4.5g
Ham – roasted	4.4g
Fish – sardines – tinned in oil	4.3g
Goose – no skin – roasted	4.3g
Beef – liver – fried	4.2g
Duck – no skin – roasted	3.7g
Cheese – ricotta – whole milk	3.6g
Chicken – leg – no skin – roasted	3.1g

Table 3: Amount of oleic oil per 100g of food (oleic oil is the major monounsaturated oil)

Food name	Oleic fatty acid per 100g
Vegetable oil – olive	71.3g
Nuts – filbert/hazel – dried – chopped	48.0g
Vegetable oil – peanut	45.6g
Nuts – pecans – dried – halves	42.8g
Nuts – almonds – shelled – chopped	36.7g
Nuts – pistachio – dried	34.8g
Nuts – cashews – dry roasted	32.0g
Bacon – broiled/fried/grilled	29.4g
Vegetable oil – corn	24.6g
Nuts – Brazil – dried – shelled	21.8g
Seeds – sesame – dried – whole	21.1g
Nuts – peanuts – spanish – dried	21.1g
Seeds – pumpkin/squash – dried	16.8g
Lamb – chop – lean/fat – broiled	13.6g
Vegetable oil – safflower	11.9g
Avocado – raw	10.2g
Nuts – walnuts	9.8g
Seeds – sunflower – dried	9.5g
Cream – whipping – heavy	9.3g
Milk – whole – dry	9.1g

Food name	Oleic fatty acid per 100g
Cheese –cream	8.6g
Hamburger – beef – 21% fat	8.2g
Cheese – parmesan – grated	7.7g
Cheese – cheddar	7.6g
Olives – green – pickled	7.5g
Pork – chop – lean – broiled/grilled	5.5g
Beef – liver – fried	4.1g
Veal – cutlet – med fat – broiled/grilled	4.0g
Egg – whole – raw – large	4.0g
Cereal – wheat germ – toasted	3.3g
Roast beef – lean/fat	3.2g
Rice – brown – long – cooked – hot	3.0g
Fish – sardines – tinned in oil	2.9g
Cheese – ricotta – whole milk	2.9g
Turkey – light/dark – no skin	2.6g
Lamb – leg – lean – roasted	2.5g

Sources of polyunsaturated fats

Any unsaturated fat with two or more double bonds is called polyunsaturated. Vegetables, nuts and seeds are the best sources.

Table 4: Amount of polyunsaturated fat per 100g of food (all polyunsaturated fats)

Food name	Polyunsaturated fat per 100g
Vegetable oil – safflower	74.3g
Vegetable oil – corn	58.7g
Nuts – walnuts	39.2g
Seeds – sunflower – dried	32.7g
Vegetable oil – peanut	32.0g
Nuts – Brazil – dried – shelled	24.1g
Seeds – sesame – dried – whole	21.8g
Seeds – pumpkin/squash – dried	20.9g

Food name	Polyunsaturated fat per 100g
Nuts – pecans – dried – halves	16.8g
Nuts – peanuts – spanish – dried	15.5g
Nuts – almonds – shelled – chopped	10.9g
Vegetable oil – olive	8.4g
Nuts – cashews – dry roasted	7.8g
Nuts – pistachio – dried	7.3g
Cereal – wheat germ – toasted	6.5g
Nuts – filbert/hazel – dried – chopped	6.0g
Bacon – pork – broiled/fried/grilled	5.8g
Fish – sardines – tinned in oil	3.4g
Cereal – 100% bran	2.8g
Seaweed – spirulina – dried	2.1g
Avocado – raw	2.0g
Chicken – leg – no skin – roasted	2.0g
Pork – chop – lean – broiled/grilled	1.9g
Goose – no skin – roasted	1.5g
Beef – liver – fried	1.5g
Egg – whole – raw – large	1.4g
Turkey – light/dark – no skin	1.4g
Duck – no skin – roasted	1.4g
Ham – reg – roasted – pork	1.4g
Cream – whipping – heavy	1.4g
Cheese – cream	1.3g
Nuts – macadamia – dried	1.3g
Egg – duck – whole – fresh – raw	1.2g
Lamb – chop – lean/fat – broiled/grilled	1.1g
Flour – corn – sifted	1.0g
Cheese – cheddar	0.9g

Good food sources of linoleic acid (the double bonded dietary essential oil)

1. Green leafy vegetables
   Kale
   Spring greens
   Swiss chard
2. Raw nuts and seeds
   Sesame
   Sunflower

    Almonds
    Flax seeds (Linseeds)

3. Meats
    Liver
    Kidneys
    Brains
    Sweetbreads

Table 5: Amount of linoleic acid per 100g of food

Food name	Linoleic acid per 100g
Vegetable oil – safflower	73.4g
Vegetable oil – corn	57.3g
Nuts – walnuts	35.2g
Vegetable oil – peanut	31.0g
Seeds – sunflower – dried	30.0g
Nuts – Brazil – dried – shelled	25.0g
Seeds – sesame – dried – whole	23.3g
Seeds – pumpkin/squash – dried	19.6g
Nuts – pecans – dried – halves	16.9g
Nuts – peanuts – spanish – dried	14.2g
Nuts – pistachio – dried	10.2g
Nuts – almonds – shelled – chopped	9.8g
Vegetable oil – olive	8.2g
Nuts – filbert/hazel – dried – chopped	6.3g
Bacon – pork – broiled/fried/grilled	5.6g
Cereal – wheat germ – toasted	5.0g
Popcorn – popped – plain	3.3g
Nuts – cashews – dry roasted	3.2g
Cornmeal – unbolted – dry	2.0g
Avocado – raw	1.7g
Lamb – chop – lean/fat – broiled/grilled	1.3g
Turkey – light/dark – no skin	1.3g
Pork – chop – lean – broiled/grilled	1.2g
Egg – whole – raw – large	1.2g
Beef – liver – fried	1.1g
Cream – whipping – heavy	0.8g
Flour – whole wheat – stirred	0.8g

Food name	Linoleic Acid per 100g
Milk – whole – dry	0.8g
Cheese – cream	0.7g
Beef – heart – lean – braised	0.7g
Olives – green – pickled	0.6g
Nuts – coconut – raw –shredded	0.6g
Fish – sardines – tinned in oil	0.6g
Cheese – cheddar	0.6g
Hamburger – beef – 21% fat	0.5g
Veal – cutlet – med fat – broiled/grilled	0.5g

Table 6: Percentages of linoleic acid

Unrefined vegetable oil	Percentages of linoleic acid
Safflower	78
Sunflower	69
Corn	62
Soya	61
Walnut	59
Cottonseed	54
Sesame	43
Rice bran	32
Peanut	31
Flax seed (Linseed)	19–22
Olive	15
Coconut	2

Unrefined oils:
- should not be subjected to temperatures above 140 degrees. Centigrade during manufacture or cooking.
- should be stored in a light proof container.
- should be consumed within 3 months of manufacture.
- should be stored in dark cool place.

Table 7: Good food sources of linolenic acid (the triple bonded dietary essential oil)

Food source	Percentages of linolenic acid
Linseeds (Flax)*	49–52
Pumpkin seeds	15
Soya oil	3–9
Walnut oil	<1
Dark green vegetables	<1

*Since linseed (flax) oil contains both dietary essential oils, it is without a doubt, the best food source of the essential fatty acids.

Table 8: Amino acids in linseed

Linseed (flax) is a premium food because of its many other nutrients. This table shows the level of amino acids per 100g of seeds.

Amino acid	g/100g
Aspartic	9.8
Threonine(*)	4.0
Serine	4.9
Glutamic	22.0
Proline	4.1
Glycine	6.4
Alanine	4.8
Cysteine	1.3
Valine(*)	5.0
Methionine(*)	0.4
Isoleucine(*)	4.3
Leucine(*)	6.7
Tyrosine	2.4
Phenylalanine(*)	4.8
Lysine(*)	4.3
Histidine(*)	2.2
Arginine	11.2

*Indicates a dietary essential amino acid.

(*Source: Personal correspondence from Paul Stitt showing an analysis performed by Doctor's Data, Chicago.*)

Table 9: Minerals in linseed

Linseed (flax) is also an excellent source of many minerals.

Element	Parts per million
Nickel	1.2
Beryllium	0.025
Calcium	2466.
Magnesium	3282.
Sodium	259.
Potassium	15319.
Copper	7.
Zinc	250.
Iron	178.
Manganese	81.20
Chromium	1.06
Cobalt	0.26
Lithium	0.269
Molybdenum	0.94
Phosphorus	5363.
Selenium	0.49
Silicon	7.
Vanadium	0.33
Sulphur	1987.
Strontium	6.2
Barium	2.3
Boron	34.1
Zirconium	0.33

Levels of toxic minerals depend upon farming methods and location. A non-organic analysis gave these readings:

Element	Parts per million
Lead	<1
Mercury	<0.1
Arsenic	0.1
Cadmium	0.3
Aluminium	7

(*Source: Personal correspondence from Paul Stitt showing an analysis performed by Doctor's Data.*)

Table 10: Other fatty acids in linseeds (flax)

Fatty acids	
8:0	Caprylic
10:0	Capric
12:0	Lauric
14:0	Myristic
14:1	Myristoleic
15:0	Pentadecanoic
15:1	Pentadecenoic
16:0	Palmitic
16:1	Palmitoleic
17:0	Heptadecanoic
17:1	Heptadecenoic
18:0	Stearic
18:1	Oleic
18:2	Linoleic
18:3	Linolenic
20:0	Arachidic

Table 11: Plant sources of gamma linolenic acid

A healthy body can convert linoleic acid (LA) into gamma linolenic acid (GLA). Some plants are a direct source of GLA:

Plant	Percentages (GLA)
Borage	24
GLA from algae	15
Blackcurrant*	15–19
Gooseberry	10–12
Evening primrose	2–9

*While blackcurrant supplies GLA, it also contains a potent GLA inhibitor and is not a recommended source.

The fish oils: omega-3 family

The major production of eicosapentanoic acid (EPA) comes from plankton in the cold waters of the Arctic and Antarctic oceans. Literally, EPA is nature's antifreeze, produced to allow plankton to survive very cold temperatures. The colder the water, the more EPA is produced by the plankton which becomes the food for fish. Thus, warm water fish have much less EPA. The highest concentration in fish is in the north Atlantic sardine with 18%. Salmon contain about 9% and mackerel about 5%.

Table 12: Comparison of EPA content in 3.5 ounce servings of selected fish

Fish	Milligrams of EPA
Anchovy	747
Salmon, chinook	633
Herring	606
Mackerel	585
Tuna, albacore	337
Halibut, Pacific	194
Cod, Atlantic	93
Trout, rainbow	84
Haddock	72
Swordfish	30
Red snapper	19
Sole	10

Appendix B:

Metabolic Reactions and Pathways

Fig 1: The fundamental reaction of nutrition

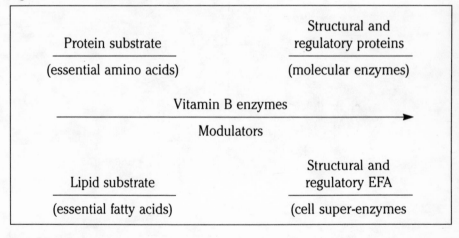

The chemical relations are shown between the essential dietary nutrients which constitute a complete set of coreactants, including protein and lipid *substrates* (the essential amino and fatty acids), *catalyst* cofactors (B vitamins) and the various *modulators*, including dietary fibre (the bowel lipid controller), the antioxidants (vitamins C and E and selenium), the lipotropes (the minor B vitamins), and the lipidic vitamins (A, D, E, K). The products consist of a variety of protein structures and regulators (enzymes) and lipid structures (e.g., the cell bilayer membrane) and regulators (e.g., prostaglandins, leukotrienes, thromboxanes).

(*Source: 1984–85 Yearbook of Nutritional Medicine, D. Rubin.*)

Fig 2: Metabolic pathway showing how the essential oil, linoleic acid (LA) is converted into other required fatty acids.

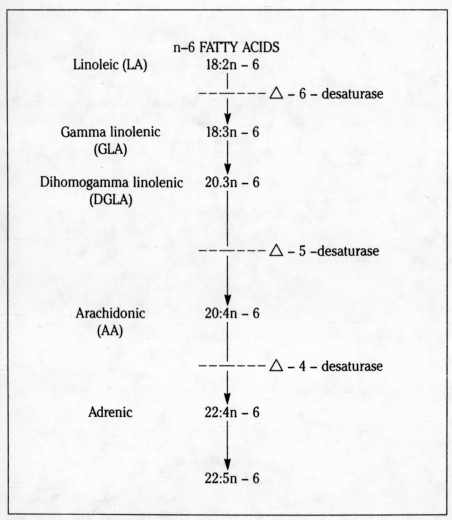

Fig 3: Metabolic pathway showing how the anti-inflammatory prostaglandin E1 is made from the essential oil – linoleic acid

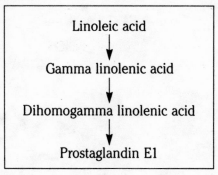

Fig 4: Metabolic pathway showing how the inflammatory prostaglandin E2 is made from the essential oil – linoleic acid

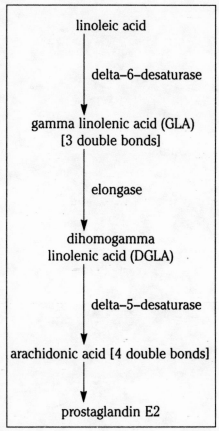

Fig 5: Metabolic pathway showing how the essential oil, alpha-linolenic acid (ALA) is converted into two required oils: (EPA) and finally (DHA)

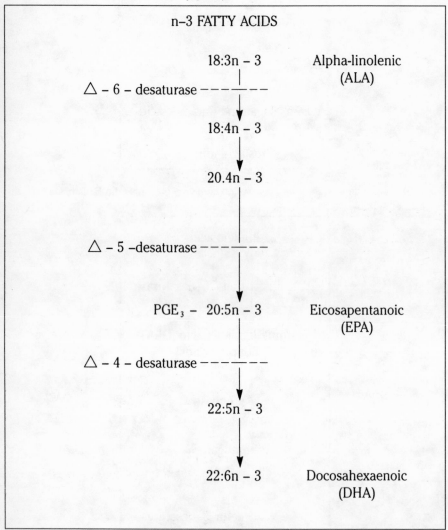

n–3 FATTY ACIDS

18:3n – 3   Alpha-linolenic (ALA)

$\triangle$ – 6 – desaturase ————

18:4n – 3

20.4n – 3

$\triangle$ – 5 –desaturase ————

PGE_3 – 20:5n – 3   Eicosapentanoic (EPA)

$\triangle$ – 4 – desaturase ————

22:5n – 3

22:6n – 3   Docosahexaenoic (DHA)

Fig 6: Metabolic pathway showing how the anti-inflammatory prostaglandin E3 is made from the essential oil: alpha-linolenic acid

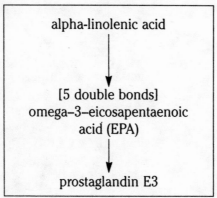

(Prostaglandin E3 opposes the action of Prostaglandin E2.)

Fig 7: Arachidonic acid conversion to prostanoids

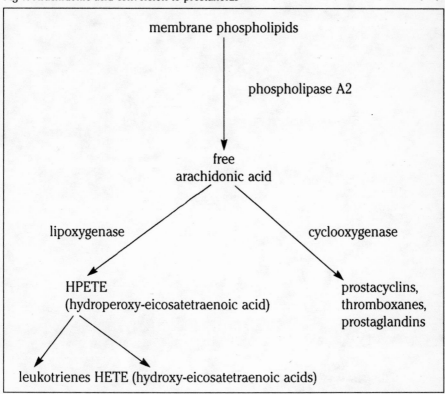

Fig 8: Leukotriene generation

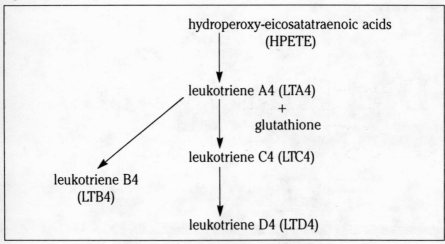

Appendix C:

Diet Analysis and Food Fat Percentages

Computer evaluation of diet

The best way to gain an understanding of what percentage of your food is fat, is to keep a diary of your food intake for one week.

After one week, the total consumption is fed into a computer, which analyses your diet and gives a complete profile of fatty acids, vitamins, minerals and amino acids.

It is essential to keep accurate information on the exact quantity of each food and drink consumed as well as how it was prepared, fried, boiled, baked, or raw.

The more sophisticated programmes allow one to change items on the spot to alter what happens to the profile when foods are changed or substituted. This allows one to make the most efficient and favourable changes to the diet.

Such programmes are readily available through many nutritional counselling and fitness centres.

Fig 1: Food fat percentages

More than 90%	Whipped cream, pork sausage, cooking oils, margarine, butter, gravy, mayonnaise
More than 80%	Spare ribs, cream cheese, salad dressing
More than 70%	Peanuts, hot dogs, pork chops, cheddar cheese, sirloin steak, bacon, lamb chops, pecans, macadamia nuts
More than 60%	Potato chips/crisps, ham, eggs, minced beef
More than 50%	Round steak, pot roast, creamed soups, ice cream
More than 40%	Whole milk, cake, doughnuts, chips/french fries
More than 30%	Muffins, chicken, biscuits, fruit pie, creamed cottage cheese, tuna fish, low-fat milk
More than 20%	Crackers, ice milk, crab meat, beef liver, lean fish
More than 10%	Bread, pretzels
Less than 10%	Sherbet, most fruits and vegetables, egg whites, baked potato, fat free milk

Appendix D:

Minimum Daily Requirements

Fig 1: Estimated average minimum daily requirements and recommended daily allowances for the essential fatty acids

STUDY	w3–EFA		w6–EFA	
	'Healthy' (% cal)	'Unhealthy' (% cal)	'Healthy' (% cal)	'Unhealthy' (% cal)
Traditional vs. Neo-modern Diet (this study)	2%	0.4%	14%	10%
Norwegian Food Survey (peacetime vs. wartime)	>1%	0.4%	8%	5%
Norwegian Linseed Study	2%	0.4%	8%	5%
Children–India (Healthy vs. phrynoderma)	1%	0.5%	2%	1%
Jap./Am. Food Survey	2%	0.4%	6%	6%
Eskimo/Dane Food Survey	2%	1.0%	2%	5%
British Food Survey		<1.0%		<7%
Parental child	0.6%	0.1%	4%	6%
Capuchin Study (Linseed oil vs. corn oil)	2%	0.2%	10%	15%
Rat Study (Brain func.) (Soy vs. safflower oil)	1–2%	0.1%	10%	10%

Therefore: MDR (w3–EFA) = 1% of calories   RDA (w3–EFA) = 2% of calories
         MDR (w6–EFA) = 2–3% of calories   RDA (w6–EFA) = 5–10% of calories

(Source: 1984-85 Yearbook of Nutritional Medicine, D. Rubin.)

Appendix E:

Suppliers of Nutritional Fat Products

Biocare Ltd
17 Pershore Road South
Kings Norton
Birmingham
B30 3EE

Advanced Nutrition Limited
8 Chilston Road
Tunbridge Wells
Kent

Spectrum Natural VegOmega 3
133 Copeland Street
Petaluma, Ca.
94952 USA

Index